The Ernst & Young Information Management Series

Information Technology for Integrated Health Systems

Also from Ernst & Young

The Ernst & Young Business Plan Guide, Second Edition
The Ernst & Young Guide to Financing for Growth
The Ernst & Young Personal Financial Planning Guide
The Name of the Game: The Business of Sports
Managing Information Strategically (The Ernst & Young
   Information Management Series)
Development Effectiveness: Strategies for IS Organizational
   Transitions (The Ernst & Young Information Management
   Series)
Privatization: Investing in State-Owned Enterprises Around the
   World
The Ernst & Young Almanac and Guide to U.S. Business Cities: 65
   Leading Places to Do Business
The Ernst & Young Guide to Total Cost Management
The Complete Guide to Special Event Management
Mergers and Acquisitions, Second Edition
Understanding and Using Financial Data: An Ernst & Young Guide
   for Attorneys

Forthcoming from Ernst & Young

(Titles subject to change)

Strategies for Accelerating the Information Systems Delivery
   Process
Holistic Management
After Reengineering: Translating Change into Improved
   Profitability

The Ernst & Young Information Management Series

Information Technology for Integrated Health Systems

Positioning for the Future

**Editors Kerry Kissinger and
Sandra Borchardt**
The Ernst & Young Boston Office

John Wiley & Sons, Inc.
New York • Chichester • Brisbane • Toronto • Singapore

This publication is designed to provide accurate and
authoritative information in regard to the subject
matter covered. It is sold with the understanding that
the publisher is not engaged in rendering legal, accounting,
or other professional services. If legal advice or other
expert assistance is required, the services of a competent
professional person should be sought.

Library of Congress Cataloging-in-Publication Data:

ISBN 0-471-11452-9

Printed in the United States of America

10 9 8 7 6 5 4 3 2 1

This book is dedicated to our health care clients, from whom we learn every day; to our fellow Ernst & Young health care consultants who picked up the slack while we were attending to this book; to Sandra Borchardt, who was the prime mover in getting the book completed on schedule; and to Janice Kissinger for her infinite patience.

K. K.

To my family: Gary and Matthew; Mom and Dad; Roxie; Becky and Tim; Randy, Anne, Keely, Corine, and Brett; Helen, Rod, and Frances; and Edward and Melissa for their patience and unconditional love and support.

S. B.

Contents

Preface

I installed my first patient accounting system in 1964. The computerized billing system utilized removable disk files to store patient demographic information, and detailed charges were entered by keying them onto punched cards. There were no terminals attached to the system, and there was no ability to inquire into account status, except through the computer console, a bouncing-ball typewriter capable of the blistering speed of 15 characters per second.

Patient bills were automatically prorated by insurance plans and were printed out in batches on the line printer. In many respects the computer, an IBM 1440 (International Business Machines), was similar to a personal computer, though quite a bit larger and significantly less powerful. The main memory was 16 kilobits and each removable disk pack held 2.4 million characters. The system had two disk drives so data could be backed up.

The installation represented a conversion from a punched-card tabulating system. Individual charges still needed to be keypunched from requisition slips that had been manually coded by the fulfilling department and fed to the computer through a card reader. Medicare was a gleam in Lyndon Johnson's eye. The billing program had been written by programmers (systems engineers) at IBM and was distributed free to hospitals that leased or purchased the 1440.

By 1965 there were 15 to 20 hospitals in the country utilizing the system, and the data processing managers from these institutions began meeting informally to share ideas about how to best utilize the system and software. They also commiserated about how many bugs they had to cope with and how slow IBM was to fix them. This informal group of hospitals became the nucleus for ECHO, which stood for Electronic Computing–Hospital Oriented, the first health care computer users' group.

As an early member of ECHO, I saw it grow and change over the years. There were two conferences held each year; over time the group grew to attract as many as 1,200 attendees—with multiple tracks, special-interest groups, and an international contingent—at venues like the Hotel del Coronado in San Diego.

ECHO's educational programs had always been very mainframe oriented, and by the late 1980s the organization waned in popularity. Its life cycle followed that of mainframe computing, and the organization, influenced by IBM, clung to a mainframe mentality far too long. The group is now extinct.

My participation in ECHO spanned 25 years. During that time the computer industry and health care organizations' use of computers changed significantly, but not radically. The IBM 1440 was called a second-generation computer by virtue of its transistorized circuitry, as opposed to the vacuum tube computers it replaced. The next generation of computers would be capable of multiprocessing, or doing several different tasks concurrently, including providing on-line access via cathode-ray tube display terminals.

Each decade has spawned a new generation of hardware and software platforms capable of doing more things at lower unit cost than its predecessor. The tools of the trade and the technology continue to advance in terms of price, performance, and ease of use. The current watchword is client-server computing, whereby computing is distributed between a relational data base stored on the server and intelligent workstations on the desktop, the client. In terms of the skill sets required to succeed with this new technology, it borders on radical change.

I have been fortunate to observe these generational changes, but I have also been struck by how much each new generation of users struggles with learning how to deploy the technology. The patient accounting system I implemented in 1964 took eight months to complete. It had significant payback for the hospital. The number of machine operators was cut in half. Bills were produced sooner, and the ability of the system to do insurance proration resulted in fewer clerical personnel and improved cash flow. The new computer was far more reliable than the machines its replaced and significantly less costly to maintain.

A recent patient accounting system implementation took two years to complete and employed the skills and efforts of a 35-person project team. Everything about the project was more complex than prior generations. The regulatory environment, the number of interfaces to other systems, the new software and operating system, the network requirements, the testing and data conversion, the procedural changes and training requirements, and coping with a new set of vendors were all complex and costly elements to deal with.

The risks and costs were significant and the rewards were difficult to measure. The most compelling reason for making the change was that the current system had become too difficult, costly, and unstable to maintain and had to be replaced. It was not return on investment that drove the decision, it was simply viewed as a necessary cost of doing business. The hospital had dug itself into a deep hole and could not get out any other way. Unfortunately, this scenario is more the norm than the exception in health care today. Many health care organizations have relied heavily on vendors for support and become locked into rigid systems designed almost entirely to meet the needs of acute-care hospitals. Executives see little value from and have much dissatisfaction with management information systems (MIS) department output. Without demonstrable value, funding shrinks. MIS staffs become weakened by tight budgetary constraints. And the hole slowly deepens.

This book is written for anyone who has a stake in the future success of information technology in health care. It was conceived to help organizations set a direction that is specific to their needs and to implement appropriate solutions successfully. It represents the collective thinking of some of the most knowledgeable people in the field today and is the culmination of over 200 years of collective experience. It describes a way of guiding the deployment of information technology assets and provides many useful tools for supporting information processes. It will give the reader a sufficient understanding of all the factors that influence a successful outcome so that he or she may proceed with confidence. Today, more than at any time in recent history, health care executives' effectiveness in dealing with this subject will determine their success or failure.

KERRY KISSINGER

Boston, Massachusetts

Acknowledgments

Our authors, listed alphabetically, are responsible for writing or contributing to the chapters indicated:

Sandra Borchardt, Senior Manager in our Boston office, oversees the general financial systems practice for our New England Health Care group.
    Chapter 8: Implementation Planning

Pam Carlson, Manager in our Chicago office, provides consulting services to our health care clients.
    Chapter 6: Technology—Architecture and Enablement (Contributor)

Kenneth R. Gebhart, Manager in our Washington, D.C., office, focuses his health care efforts on information technology, process innovation, and organization change management. (kenneth.gebhart@ey.com)
    Chapter 7: The People Part (Contributor)

Randy M. Golob, Manager in our Minneapolis office, specializes in strategic technology planning for multientity health care systems. (randy.golob@ey.com)
    Chapter 1: The Strategic Context (Contributor)
    Chapter 3: Reengineering the Process
    Chapter 6: Technology—Architecture and Enablement

Patricia S. Heller, Partner in our Boston office, has extensive experience with the development and implementation of computerized health care information systems in both the clinical and financial areas. (patricia.heller@ey.com)
    Chapter 4: Assessing Your Strengths (Contributor)

Kerry Kissinger, Partner in our Boston office and Area Director for Health Care Information Technology Consulting in the Northeast, delivers professional services to the health care industry. (kerry.kissinger@ey.com)
    Chapter 1: The Strategic Context
    Chapter 9: Tying it Together

Deborah T. Maslia, Senior Manager in our Atlanta office, specializes in health care financial systems implementation. (deborah.maslia@ey.com)
    Chapter 2: Developing a Vision

Daniel S. Nutkis, Director of our National Practice of Health Care Technology, has extensive experience in areas relating to health information networks. (daniel.nutkis@ey.com)
    Chapter 6: Technology—Architecture and Enablement (Contributor)

Edward P. Phelan, Senior Manager in our Hartford office, is responsible for directing the performance improvement consulting practice in Connecticut.
    Chapter 3: Reengineering the Process (Contributor)

John F. Quinn, Principal in our National Health Care Information Services, has an extensive background in information systems planning, development, support, and systems integration. John is also Technical Committee Chairman of the HL7 Health Care Information Standards Organization. (john.quinn@ey.com)
Chapter 5: Emerging Standards

Patrick J. Rossignol, Ph.D., Partner in our New York office and National Director of Ernst & Young's Health Care Information Systems Planning Practice, has assisted health care providers in a variety of engagements including information systems planning and software selection and implementation.
Chapter 5: Emerging Standards (Contributor)

Marilyn M. San Clemente, Manager in our Boston office, has assisted health care clients with systems planning, software selection, and all phases of software implementation. (marilyn.san-clemente@ey.com)
Chapter 4: Assessing Your Strengths

Jeffrey P. Tarte, Partner based in our Charlotte office, is co-director of our Northeast Region Integrated Service Delivery to Managed Care Organizations.
Chapter 7: The People Part

Jay E. Toole, Partner in our Atlanta office and National Director of Ernst & Young's Health Care Information Technology Consulting Practice, is responsible for planning and delivering information systems services to the firm's health care clients. (jay.toole@ey.com)
Chapter 2: Developing a Vision

We would like to thank our Ernst & Young colleagues who have read or reviewed parts of this book and those who supported the process by allowing the authors time away from client work to complete their chapters. We would also like to thank the

Boston Health Care Administrative staff, especially Jo'Anne O'Brien, Michele LaCerda, Ann Weld, Laura McMaster, Caroline DePina, and Nicole Goguen for their efforts with the manuscript and graphics production. And without the heroic efforts of Elizabeth Breiner and Elizabeth Macdonald, we would have never made the publisher's deadline.

Special thanks to Jan Roehl-Anderson and Sheck Cho for providing this opportunity and to the authors' families, for without their patient support and understanding, the book would have never been written.

Finally, thanks to Jon Zonderman for taking the contributions of many individuals and turning them into a book, for his constant support and encouragement, and for his subject-matter contributions. And thanks to Tracy King-Astwood, our editor at John Wiley & Sons, for her patience and perseverance.

SANDRA BORCHARDT

Boston, MA

The Strategic Context

On December 20, 1994, the *Wall Street Journal* carried a front-page story about the impending financial failure of a Health Care International (HCI) hospital in Clydebank, Scotland. The $280 million, 260-bed hospital and adjoining 168-room four-star hotel had opened only six months earlier.

The project was designed and built with the goal of being an international tertiary-care center with leading surgeons and state-of-the-art technology and with systems such as a biplane peripheral angiography laboratory, linear accelerators for radiation therapy, and ambulatory surgical rooms with portable fluoroscopy. The hospital was also considered on the cutting edge of information technology because of a paperless information system. But as of December most of the beds were still empty. The flood of patients from southern Europe, northern Africa, and the Middle East never materialized, and the hospital has been forced by its creditors into the British equivalent of bankruptcy proceedings. Top management has been dismissed and many original investors will see their stakes completely wiped out.

The problem the hospital experienced lies not with the quality of care—mortality and morbidity rates were very low for the small number of patients who actually used the facility—but with the strategy of the project's founders, who believed that if they invested heavily in technology and world-class talent, they would attract the volume of paying patients needed to offset the debt and generate a sizable profit. Not only did this strategy miss the mark, but it has also resulted in millions of dollars in lost investments by such investors as the Harvard University Endowment Fund and Montgomery Medical Ventures, a venture-capital affiliate of Montgomery Securities in San Francisco.

The strategy of HCI is representative of the strategy many hospital administrators in the United States have taken in the past—investing in systems and technology with the objective of swaying physician preferences and increasing referrals and volumes. Although this may have had some positive results in the past, in and of itself the strategy is no longer valid today because of the numerous changes in the marketplace—mainly the increased competition in health care and the increased number of educated buyers who purchase health care based on cost as well as quality.

The health care industry in the United States is today undergoing a massive economic triage. The balance of power has shifted from providers to payers, and the payers are pushing patients into lower-cost care settings and patterns of treatment. As this thrust to lower costs intensifies, providers are responding creatively and are creating a huge shift in the available sites of care, more closely matching patients' acuity with the level of care.

The push for health care reform—both at the national level and in many states—has left an indelible and irreversible imprint on the landscape of the health care system. What began in the nineteenth century as a charitable, community-based effort to care for the sick and needy has evolved to become a very large and complex industry. Since shortly after World War II, its growth has been fueled by government spending, mostly at the federal level.

Federal funds first paid for bricks and mortar (Hill-Burton in the 1950s) and then for implementation of the Great Society programs (Medicare and Medicaid in the 1960s), which broadened access to health care and assured providers that they would be virtually free of bad debts. More recently federal support for medical schools and academic medical centers has doubled the output of physicians per year over the decade of the 1970s. The trajectory of the spending curve was so robust that the Health and Human Services Department projected a crash in the form of a bankrupt Medicare Trust Fund by the year 2000.

This prompted a major shift in thinking and policy, and the 1980s saw reimbursement for health care services shift from a cost-plus formula to a fixed fee for service paid prospectively. By the mid-1980s, hospitals were at risk financially if they couldn't render care cost-effectively. But their problems had only just begun.

The handwriting has been on the wall for providers for the past decade. The handwriting reads something like this: If the federal and state governments are the largest source of revenues for hospitals and physicians (and they are cutting back on the share they are willing and able to pay), then providers have to raise the prices they charge to others in order to keep up with the demand and the high costs of technology. In other words, they have to shift more of the costs from the public sector to the private sector, which provides insurance coverage for its employees.

To paraphrase Lee Iacocca, there're more sutures in a Dodge than there's steel, meaning that health insurance for workers who make Dodge cars costs Chrysler more than the steel that goes into the cars. So now everybody's on the cost-containment bandwagon, and they are incenting or directing patients to the lowest cost site or modality of care.

Large corporate employers are coming to realize that controlling health care costs is becoming a critical factor in their own competitiveness and overall financial success. They have watched health care costs rise over the years to become a significant percentage of their total expenses. In 1993, for example, total health benefits costs averaged 9.8 percent of payroll expenses and 11.1 percent of payroll for employers with more than 500 workers, according to Foster-Higgins, the New York-based benefits consulting firm.

With no relief in sight, employers have taken it upon themselves to intercede in the process and attempt to slow health care inflation by inflicting some level of competition into the health care marketplace. These efforts are proving effective and are resulting in dramatic changes in the way the health care industry operates as well as in the way health care executives use information technology.

Health care organizations can only succeed in this newly cost-competitive environment if they refocus on the needs and demands of the customer. For health insurance plans the customer is the employer or individual who is purchasing the insurance; for providers the financial customer is increasingly the health insurance plan, and the customer for quality and access is the individual plan member—the patient.

Customers, whether financial, quality, or access oriented, are becoming more educated and more involved. They are basing their buying decisions on bottom-line cost and on quality as defined by outcomes information, not on whether the hospital has a biplane peripheral angiography laboratory, a linear accelerator for radiation therapy, or an ambulatory surgery room with portable fluoroscopy.

Specialists are losing business to primary-care physicians; nursing homes are being challenged by home health care; and acute-care hospitals are shrinking as subacute hospitals and day-surgery centers are proliferating.

As a provider, it is difficult to know who your friends are. Yet in most markets, it won't be possible to survive into the twenty-first century as a solo or stand-alone entity. The acute-care hospital has become the mainframe of health care and is rapidly losing its position as the center of care. It is becoming a cost center in a larger network of services, and it must compete on the basis of value. Lower-cost providers offering similar services will continue to capture patient volume at the expense of less efficient providers. Providers will continue to consolidate into integrated health systems that can match the right level of care with the needs of patients and their families.

As the financial risks continue to shift from the payers to the providers, providers need to better understand and control the costs associated with treating patients. And they increasingly need to effect this cost control over many caregiving settings.

Just as important as controlling costs is the ability to demonstrate value. In this case, value means positive outcomes of treatment or lower incidence of illness, or both. Quality of care will be as much a function of teamwork among caregivers as it now is a function of the skills of the individual caregiver.

Cross-functional teams are increasingly being formed to focus on a patient's needs across sites of care. This is often described as a seamless approach to patient care.

The Role of Technology

A variety of technologies are being considered to achieve cost and quality goals. Many of them involve heroic life-saving or life-extending support systems for the very young and the very old. Others are in some way or other aimed at diagnosing and treating the patient in the lowest cost setting.

In 1992 outpatient surgical procedures exceeded inpatient surgical procedures for the first time, and the gap continues to widen. The pressure to prevent patients from becoming hospitalized and to reduce their lengths of stay once they are hospitalized is intense. The market has forced providers into a demand and supply tailspin. In some major population centers the overcapacity of hospital beds is estimated to be 30 percent or so. We are witnessing a shift of tremendous magnitude from stand-alone hospitals to affiliations and mergers of hospitals, nursing homes, home health agencies, pharmacy operations, imaging centers, and physician groups into large regional systems of health care aimed at providing for all the needs of a given population on a fixed-capitated basis.

Implicit in this seamless approach is the ability to give caregivers access to information about diagnosis and treatment at the point of care. This information must be accurate, timely, and, above all, easily accessible. It is no wonder then that health care executives are placing increased importance on information systems and are challenging their chief information officers (CIOs) to transform their disparate, disconnected, acute-care-focused systems into deliverywide health information networks.

So what does this mean for the CIO in health care today? Is there any hope for getting out of the current information towers of Babel?

The good news, from an information systems perspective, is that the health care industry is fast becoming less regulated, more competitive, and less fragmented. It is in the process of redeploying its resources to focus more on the resulting outcomes for patients, higher levels of service to their families, and lower costs to their health plan.

Competing this way represents a 180-degree turn from the old way of doing business under a straight indemnity fee-for-service model. Under that model, hospitals and other health care facilities compete for a referral base and aim to meet the needs of physicians who control the referral population. Large institutions saw as their customers the referring physicians and neglected the needs of other stakeholders: the health plan, which wants lower costs; the individual being served, who wants easy access and a simplified visit process; even the nursing staff, who want more time to spend with patients.

Therein lies the frustration with information technology in health care institutions. The value of information technology is dramatically different depending on which stakeholder is being served. And value is difficult to measure in a system that is so fractured. The misaligned goals under an indemnity-based health care system make it difficult, if not impossible, to purchase systems that meet the goals of all stakeholders because those goals vary depending on where the stakeholder is in the system (employer, member, payer, hospital, primary-care physician, staff specialist, etc.).

The only palatable solution in this environment is to implement specialized solutions that address narrowly defined needs. This type of solution, however, only compounds the frustration in information technology. Even though many departments within a hospital are automated, information technology has failed to produce the results observed in other industries. The health care industry has watched from the sidelines as other industries have leveraged information technology to produce remarkable gains and fundamentally change the way business is conducted.

Many of these frustrations will increase, however, as competition increases in the health care industry and managed care becomes the accepted way of conducting business. By refocusing on the employers and consumers as customers, the health care industry will experience some of the gains other industries have experienced through innovative uses of information technology. In the short term, however, the shift from the current fractured structure to a more aligned and cost-competitive structure will exacerbate the shortcomings of current systems. With this shift, many administrators are finding that their financial systems and patient-care systems cannot easily support new requirements and the new customer focus.

From Mainframe to Mini to Desktop

Fragmentation has also taken its toll on information systems development. The majority of hospitals rely on vendor software for their most urgent needs. Although programmer rich, few hospitals have developed the kind of in-house technical skills necessary to allow them to adopt advanced technology and layer it on top of their legacy systems in order to achieve a reasonable degree of systems integration.

In the 1960s the largest hospitals—those over 400 beds—could afford to acquire one of the mainframe systems available at that time and develop their own software for patient registration, patient billing, payroll, and other financial applications. Since only about 900 of the nearly 6,000 hospitals in the United States were large enough to go it alone, several mainframe vendors like IBM, Burroughs, Honeywell, Control Data, and National Cash Register (NCR) began software-development efforts that would allow several hospitals to share a single mainframe system. Over the following decade, several service bureau companies sprang up to service smaller hospitals.

As the price of computer technology came down, smaller hospitals could afford their own systems, particularly if they could spread the cost of software development over many hospitals. Through the 1970s the number of hospital software companies multiplied. They offered systems both for specific departments and for hospitalwide use. The personal computer revolution of the 1980s further enabled hospitals to push these systems into the smallest hospitals and small departments within hospitals.

The proliferation of hospital software firms was so great that a shakeout was inevitable. As hospitals' belts tightened in the 1980s and the personal computer continued its inexorable march onto more and more desks, the mainframe and minicomputer hospital software companies began to falter, merge, be bought out and go bankrupt. Research and development budgets shrank, and staffs and unessential products and services were cut. But through it all, the companies that did best were those that maintained a sharp focus on the needs of their hospital customers.

What was once a strength has become a weakness. The hospital software companies' focus on the needs of stand-alone hospitals with proprietary software solutions is totally out of synch with the rapidly accelerating formation of regional health care systems. Hospitals have relied so heavily on these externally developed systems that they have only minimal in-house data processing capabilities. The hospitals' data processing staffs are small, are generally stronger as programmers than as analysts, and are more familiar with applying and testing vendor modifications than with designing and developing systems. To make matters worse, hospital data processing staffs have not kept pace with technology. They have relatively little competence in managing networks, little knowledge of state-of-the-art client-server technology, and little experience with more advanced technologies such as optical imaging, pen-based computing, and object-oriented programming. They're trapped.

In addition, information technology has historically supported financial functions such as charge capture, billing, accounts receivable, accounts payable, and general ledger. It is in these areas where information technology is most mature and provides a clear advantage over manual systems. Early implementation of information systems to support these functions was driven by finance, and computer operations supporting finance fell under the umbrella of the Chief Financial Officer. The value of these systems was measured by their ability to reduce overhead, capture charges and support a lower number of days in receivables.

Many of the same measures of value for these systems apply today, and the existing information systems still meet many administrative needs. But as managed care penetration has increased, administrators are finding that their current financial systems cannot support the pricing arrangements specified in the increasing number of managed care contracts. Rather than modify legacy systems, most hospital executives are choosing to add contract management modules.

Contract management is one of the most obvious weaknesses of current financial systems. Another, more subtle, weakness is in the fundamental structure of these systems. Using the information from these systems could be misleading when trying to use the information to form strategic decisions in an increasingly competitive environment.

Health care executives have to completely reshape their organizations into systems of care, yet they don't have the information systems to support this massive restructuring. The hospital has itself become the mainframe of the health care system, and its role is changing from the center of competence and the epicenter of care to that of a cost center and just another node in a network of equally important care settings. Currently installed computer systems and support staffs mitigate against this change. Computer technology has become a disabler rather than an enabler in the implementation of strategies for affiliation and provider network development. The path out of the trap is neither quick nor easy.

Health care executives must begin to think about making major investments in information technology. Until recently, hospitals have typically spent 2 to 3 percent of their operating budgets on information systems. Manufacturing concerns have been spending 3 to 5 percent, and financial services companies have been spending 8 to 10 percent. The options for health care executives are limited. Despite the relatively modest levels of investment to date, there is significant sunk cost in current systems, some of which perform a useful function for a portion of current and future needs.

The ability to collect and disseminate information about a patient's history and current treatment across different care settings and providers is absolutely vital in today's environment.

For the most part, integrated solutions cannot be found among traditional health care software vendors. The vendors are as much locked into the past as IBM was with its mainframe mind-set. They are still about the business of providing and maintaining acute-care, fee-for-service solutions in a managed care market that is rapidly moving toward capitation.

The new requirements demand that CIOs reshape their organizations to become systems integrators capable of adopting new technologies, including such things as image processing, pen-based computing, client-server computing, multimedia workstations, interface engines, voice recognition, wireless networks, and expert systems. We'll learn more about these in later chapters. Successful health care organizations will be those that can apply these emerging technologies effectively to address business requirements.

The business requirements that characterize integrated health care networks can be translated into a new set of technology-enabled health care applications. These applications include the computer-based patient record (CPR), advanced nursing support, imaging, managed care systems, electronic data interchange (EDI) and physician/ambulatory systems.

Figure 1.1 shows the relationship between technology and its application. In reality, successful health care organizations will integrate various technologies with their business practices

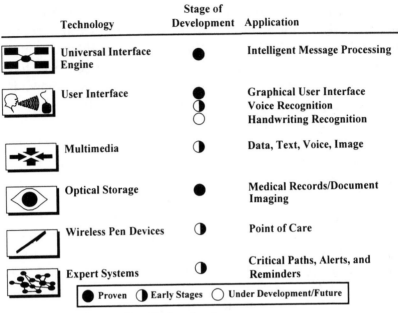

Technology	Stage of Development	Application
Universal Interface Engine	●	**Intelligent Message Processing**
User Interface	● ◑ ○	**Graphical User Interface** **Voice Recognition** **Handwriting Recognition**
Multimedia	◑	**Data, Text, Voice, Image**
Optical Storage	●	**Medical Records/Document Imaging**
Wireless Pen Devices	◑	**Point of Care**
Expert Systems	◑	**Critical Paths, Alerts, and Reminders**

● **Proven**   ◑ **Early Stages**   ○ **Under Development/Future**

Figure 1.1   *Emerging Technologies*

to lower costs, improve service levels, and enhance quality and continuity of care.

Summary

As we will see in the chapters that follow, information technology requires a shared vision of the organization, its scope, and its mission. It also requires management to take a process view of the organization, a view that crosses functional boundaries and focuses on adding value to patients and their families. It requires that CIOs objectively assess their departments' capabilities and prepare to move away from point solutions toward integrated network solutions. Along the way, the information technology function within an integrated health care system will need to become stronger and better disciplined in order to build credibility, manage expectations, and deliver timely solutions to its users.

The following are just some of the questions we will answer in this book:

- What is or should be the role of information technology? Is it a line or staff function?

- What should be the relationship between information technology and the user community?

- How should health care executives address make or buy decisions when it comes to applications software?

- Is there such a thing as a critical mass of information technology resources required in order to build your own system? What can be learned from other industries regarding this issue?

- What can be done to effectively sustain legacy systems while moving toward an enterprisewide architecture?

- How can health care executives get an organization to agree on standards and principles of operation?

- How should the information technology department be organized to deal with the current and near-future environment? What are the critical skill sets needed?

This book describes the most important steps health care executives can take to ensure that their information infrastructure supports their business strategy and plans.

2

Developing a Vision

Overview

Responding to changes in the health care industry that are increasingly integrating providers, payers, employers, patients, and other players requires health care organizations to consider not only their strategic direction and vision from the business orientation but also the ability of information technology to support and further that vision. An information technology (IT) vision consists of a specific view of the future state of the organization's information technology; this vision provides the necessary linkage among the business strategy for the entire enterprise, visions for specific processes, and technological action.

This chapter explores each component used to develop the IT vision. These components, defined below, directly affect the specifics of an IT vision and provide the guidance and direction to tailor that vision to support the business goals and strategies of each unique environment and organization. We further show that unless each component is considered in the planning process, the end result of the IT vision may be based on flawed reasoning, and the ability of the organization to justify the added expenses necessary in information technology to meet the demands of health care reform will be significantly impaired.

Components of a Vision

There are four components to the development of the IT vision, as shown in Figure 2.1.

- *Industry Trends and Directions.* What emerging forces in the health care market will influence the ultimate strategies of integrated health delivery? Examples include the formation of large purchasers of health care services and the interactions with groups of integrated providers. How do health care providers migrate from

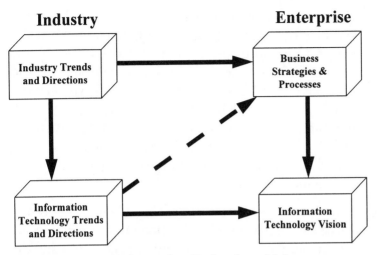

Figure 2.1 *An Information Technology Vision . . .
The Development*

a world of independent providers focused on treating
illness to one in which care is delivered and measured
against expected quality outcomes and performance?

■ *Information Technology Trends and Directions.* How
will the information systems vendors and developers
utilize advanced technologies in the market to respond
to the health care organizational and operational
needs? How can providers migrate from past information systems environments, based on financial orientation and fragmented applications, into an environment
that is clinically oriented and strongly integrated not
only between applications but also between entities
within the enterprise? Will health care be able to
leverage information tools and techniques developed in
other industries, such as banking and manufacturing?
Will these trends have a positive influence on the individual organization's strategies and directions, and enable them to more quickly take advantage of technology
in achieving a competitive advantage?

■ *Enterprise Business Strategies and Processes.* What are the specific business strategies as defined by the enterprise? These strategies are directly influenced by the nature of the business, the external environment, and future goals and directions. They should have been defined and supported by executive management. We will present a straw-man list of business strategies typically defined for an integrated delivery system and later use it to develop the information technology vision for future planning.

■ *Enterprise Information Technology Vision.* Clearly, the IT vision is influenced and defined by the components described above and, by definition, ends up being the technology vision necessary to support the individual enterprise's strategies, which have in turn been influenced by the industry's trends, directions, and information technology enablers.

Industry Trends and Directions

In developing an enterprise information technology vision, it is important to define overall industry trends that can serve as planning benchmarks. This is particularly important because the health care industry is undergoing dramatic changes as a result of reform initiatives at both the federal and state levels as well as strong market forces. To accomplish this, it is often helpful to project the state of the industry five years ahead and compare this to the current state.

Figure 2.2 provides a summary of expected changes in the health care industry by comparing future state to current state related to structure, process, and outcome. It is important to note that the pace of evolution to the future state will vary by

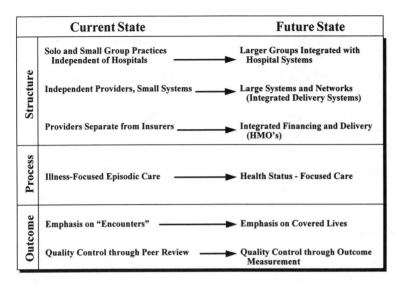

Figure 2.2   *The Health Care Industry . . . Trends and Directions*

region or locale. For instance, by mid-1995, areas such as California and greater Minneapolis already resemble what we define as the future state.

Structure

Physicians who have been organized in solo or small group practices and who have been independent of hospitals are beginning to merge into larger groups, and over time will become more fully integrated with hospital systems. This form of horizontal integration will help align the goals of the two major providers in the health care delivery system: physicians and hospitals. These integrated delivery systems—or health networks—compete with each other for managed care contracts from larger and larger purchasing groups in geographic regions. Contracts will increasingly cover the full continuum of care with a focus on reducing costs on a per-member per-month basis.

In the past, there has been a clear delineation between health care providers and health care insurers in the marketplace. Insurers were third parties who provided indemnity coverage to individuals and then paid providers for services. As the trend toward managed care continues, providers are assuming an increasing proportion of the financing risk for members or patients included in their contracts. As providers begin to offer health plans and insurers develop provider networks, we see integrated financing and delivery organizations prepared to contract directly with purchasers or employers.

Process

In the past, health care focused on treating problems or illnesses at the point where the patient showed up for treatment. The process was episodic in nature and was centered around diagnosing and treating specific problems or illnesses but was not focused on wellness or overall health status of the individual. As the industry moves toward contracted care, health care delivery organizations are implementing processes to measure and manage the health status of members, with a focus on keeping individuals healthy and out of the health care delivery system. At the same time, improved operational processes are beginning to be developed to manage the continuum of care among providers within the integrated delivery system for treatment of illnesses or diseases.

Outcomes

Another major shift in the health care industry is the movement from emphasizing market share based on number of encounters (inpatient stays, physician office visits, etc.) to market share based on covered lives. Under fee for service, providers focused on delivering more services as a measure of success. Under capitation, the number of members covered by a health plan or delivery system will be the key measure of market share.

Although initial contracts may be largely based on lowest price, as pressure continues to drive price down in the industry, quality indicators and outcomes will become important criteria for purchasers choosing health plans. In the past, quality-control efforts have been centered around peer review (e.g., physicians reviewing physicians). In the future, there will be significant emphasis on measuring outcomes and implementing quality-control techniques throughout the delivery system. Clinical protocols, or clinical guidelines, will be developed based on outcomes research and concurrence among peer physicians about what processes and techniques work best. These protocols will be built into the quality-control process of an integrated delivery system to ensure consistency throughout the organization. Use of protocols will also provide predictability in managing the cost of diagnosing and treating disease groups.

Information Technology Trends and Directions

Information technology will evolve in the health care industry to respond to industry trends and the changing industry model. Figure 2.3 provides a summary of key information-technology trends that are directly related to the trends in the health care industry overall.

Patient-Centered Orientation

In the past, health care information systems have been developed around encounters of care (inpatient days, outpatient visits, physician visits, etc.) and were largely based on collecting financial information needed to bill and collect for services. Even so-called order communication(s), or order management systems, were mostly designed to collect financial information rather than to support care-delivery processes within a hospital

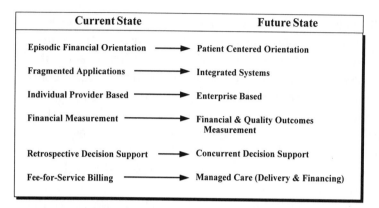

Current State	Future State
Episodic Financial Orientation ⟶	Patient Centered Orientation
Fragmented Applications ⟶	Integrated Systems
Individual Provider Based ⟶	Enterprise Based
Financial Measurement ⟶	Financial & Quality Outcomes Measurement
Retrospective Decision Support ⟶	Concurrent Decision Support
Fee-for-Service Billing ⟶	Managed Care (Delivery & Financing)

Figure 2.3   *The Health Care Industry . . . Information Technology Trends & Directions*

or other care-delivery system. In the future state, information systems will be developed with a patient-or member-centered orientation. All demographic, financial, and clinical data related to patients or members of a contracted care plan will be collected, stored, and maintained for the full continuum of care (e.g., primary-care physician to specialist to hospital, etc.), and over time will become a longitudinal or lifetime medical history.

Integrated Systems

In addition to a basic financial orientation, traditional systems were comprised of "fragmented applications." This was because most hospitals and other large providers purchased applications from multiple vendors, often operating on disparate hardware and software platforms. Point-to-point interfaces were developed between applications to allow information to be passed back and forth. Often these interfaces were poorly developed and implemented, resulting in less than optimum access to data from one application to another.

In some cases, hoping to simplify the support required, hospitals purchased applications from a single vendor. The

single-vendor concept, where one company developed all applications needed for a hospital, has not been successful for
many providers, particularly larger organizations. It has proven
to be very difficult for any single vendor to provide best-of-
breed applications in all application areas.

In the future, financial, clinical, and patient care systems
will be far more integrated, with easy access to data regardless
of the hardware or software platform. The architecture of future systems will allow for distributed data access with a common user interface for viewing and using information. Interface
engines will provide both connectivity and seamless exchange
of data, as well as tool sets to lower the cost of developing a best-
of-breed environment.

Enterprise Based

Even systems designed in the 1980s and early 1990s, which fac-
tored in a business process approach rather than a strict functional approach, were developed based on individual provider
types (e.g., hospitals, physicians, home health, etc.). Software
companies focused on one segment of the health care market
and provided capabilities to support only the business processes
of specific types of organizations. These systems were not built
to interconnect providers who have formed an integrated delivery system.

In the future, systems will be enterprise based to support
not only the requirements of each provider entity within an integrated delivery system but also to support the enterprisewide
needs. An example of such is the need to identify the patient on
an enterprisewide basis and provide a common registration and
scheduling capability, regardless of the provider location.

Financial and Quality/Outcomes Measurement

Measuring financial and operational results has always been a
key requirement for health care applications and will continue
to be critical on an enterprise basis. However, the ability to define and measure quality and outcomes is becoming increasingly

critical. Information systems in the future will need to retain large amounts of clinically significant data over time to support development of quality indicators, outcomes measures and clinical protocols or clinical guidelines. Standardization of nomenclature, coding systems, and syntax will be essential for sharing quality and outcomes data between delivery organizations.

Concurrent Decision Support

As integrated delivery systems develop and assume more financial risk, the need for decision-support data will escalate geometrically. In the past, decision-support systems were built around collecting retrospective financial, demographic, and clinical (often limited) data. This data was often put into a relational database with user-access tools for reporting. This capability will be extremely important going forward; but in addition, concurrent decision support will be required by clinicians or caregivers. The concept will be centered around providing caregivers the information they need at the time clinical decisions are made. Examples of this are alerts or reminders that are built into the system and clinical protocols based on a specific diagnosis or problem.

Managed Care

The migration from fee-for-service billing to managed care or contracted care such as capitation is an important trend. In the past, hospital- and physician-based patient accounting systems were built completely around fee-for-service billing, which has evolved to be extremely complex in the United States. These systems did not operate well in a managed care environment, and had to be enhanced in order to support managed care. As an alternative, stand-alone applications can be purchased and interfaced with a patient accounting system. Recently, managed care systems to support the insurance or financing side of the business have been developed by different software vendors. These systems, which have been used in the past by HMOs, will now be needed by integrated delivery systems that establish their own health plans.

New Technologies

Health care applications developed in the past provided limited flexibility and support to end users. This lack of user-friendliness made it more difficult for individuals to significantly change operational processes that depended on information technology. This led to poorly installed systems and limited tangible benefits. New health care applications are incorporating emerging technologies that enable users to change business processes. Examples include graphical user interface (GUI), voice and handwriting recognition, multimedia workstations, imaging, wireless handheld computers, and expert systems. These technologies will support all of the previously described technological trends.

Graphical User Interface

The GUI is a windows-based environment on a personal computer, or PC, a workstation that allows the user to easily open files and navigate through applications. Use of a common user interface such as Microsoft Windows, which has been adopted by most health care software vendors, enhances an organization's ability to train users and install new applications. It also supports improved work flows.

Recognition

Voice and handwriting recognition are emerging technologies that could provide an easy way for physicians and other care-givers to input data into a system. Voice-recognition software can be taught to recognize and understand an individual voice in conversational English and will respond to voice commands for inputting and processing data. Handwriting recognition is a similar technology that can be taught to software. Both of these are now being used in selected health care applications.

Multimedia

Multimedia allows you to display or play back multiple forms of information, including data and text, voice, image, and video, on one PC or workstation. Virtually all new health care applications centered around the computer-based patient record are being developed by software vendors using multimedia.

Imaging

Imaging technology can be used to input and store documents as well as radiological or medical images. A common application for document imaging is medical records. Although document imaging does not capture discrete data elements (it only captures an image of the document), it may become an effective transition strategy to an electronic medical record, allowing information captured manually to be integrated with information entered electronically to form a totally computerized patient file.

Medical imaging has only been implemented in a relatively small number of medical centers in the country due to the high cost of implementation and operation. As costs drop and telemedicine becomes more popular, medical imaging may provide significant leverage to extend the reach of tertiary-care providers and may reduce the costs of medical education.

Point-of-Service Technology

Ease of data entry and documentation (at the patient's bedside, the physician's exam room, etc.) will be an essential requirement for development of the computer-based patient record. Handheld devices are one means of accomplishing this task. These devices will be tailored to the individual caregiver and will support care planning, delivery, and documentation. They will communicate over a wireless network to other computers to process and store data. Point-of-care devices have already been developed in health care to support nurses at the bedside and home health caregivers who travel to the patient's location.

Expert Systems

Expert systems provide the capability to apply an established set of rules (developed by experts) to a specific situation (e.g., an individual patient). For example, expert systems could be used to assist a physician in diagnosing a problem and prescribing a treatment plan. They could also be used to alert or notify the physician immediately when certain clinically significant factors occur. A simple example of this would be the ability to check for drug-to-drug interaction for an individual based on active drug dosage and expert rules on interaction.

Enterprise Business Strategies and Processes

The previous sections focused on the environmental considerations important in the visioning process. The next two sections discuss the particulars of an individual enterprise's business and technology trends.

With so many factors influencing the ultimate IT vision and with so much riding on the final decisions regarding scarce resources, what tools can be used to define the vision? How can an organization ensure that when it reaches its final destination, it has executive management buy in and the IT vision is based on actual environmental and organizational factors currently being faced or will be faced in the future?

Although each component of the visioning exercise will require special attention and multiple iterations in development and implementation, there are some basic steps helpful in the definition of each component.

1. *Clearly define the enterprise model* of the future organization. Who will the key players be, and what organizational and process changes are expected? How will each entity that is part of the enterprise be connected to the central organization (i.e., financial, clinical, organizational, and reporting), and what will the impact be of competitors? These questions need to be

revisited often, since the pace of acquisitions and ventures is difficult to keep up with, and the results of such organizational changes can be very significant in the information technology planning process.

2. *Conduct a series of workshops* or facilitated sessions that get increasingly specific as you near the definition of the IT vision. Sessions should contain a manageable number of individuals who are key to the specific component under study. For example, the facilitated sessions to define organizational strategies might include key management individuals who are most influential in moving the organization into the next stage of strategic development and goal realization. On the other hand, the IT visioning exercise might include some of the same key management individuals involved in organizational strategic planning but may also include specific information technology representatives with technical skills to allow more specific and realistic visioning.

3. *Use traditional tools* to help define each component. These include consideration of goals, objectives, critical success factors, key stakeholders and competitors, and SWOT (strengths, weaknesses, opportunities, and threats) analysis. These tools will help uncover some of the key factors that will have an impact on the final IT vision.

4. *Consult with customers* in each area to understand key issues for the current and future environments. For example, to help understand the organizational strategies, speak with the physicians or key payers and managed care teams to understand their current and future needs from the organization.

5. *Employ experts in all fields* of the health care industry and health care technology, and use benchmarks to

assess the best practices in information technology for understanding the scope of alternatives and examples of innovation that exist not only inside the health care industry but also, especially, those outside this traditional provider-oriented industry.

With the evolution of integrated delivery systems, enterprisewide processes must be closely reviewed and evaluated in light of the technology implementations to support these processes. This will help avoid the risk of being left with "silos" of operations that lead the IT vision in directions not beneficial for the integrated environment. After these processes have been redesigned or reengineered to improve effectiveness and efficiencies, the information technology vision will have a very different flavor from a vision designed to support the functionally rigid organization.

Enterprise Strategy Definition

After the *future-state vision of the industry* has been examined by the organization and information technology alternatives are understood, the next step in defining the enterprise's ultimate IT vision is to understand and clarify the enterprise's current and future business strategies.

The following section presents a model of a specific organization's business strategies—one we think will come very close to defining your particular strategies, given the current state of the industry and reform implications. This model is derived from and influenced by many factors including the industry future-state vision—focused on integrated delivery systems. Additionally, this model will drive the definition of an information technology vision tailored for your organization.

By defining the enterprise's business strategies, you can start to understand not only the resulting IT vision, but also the vision of what will be needed in information systems production and management to meet and support the migration of where you are today as a business to where you want to be tomorrow. How will you use information technology to gain competitive advantage and to capture the information needed to manage your organization into the twenty-first century? Figure 2.4 presents the straw-man model of a specific organization's business strategies.

Such strategies may be formally defined in a strategic planning project conducted by executive management, with or without the support of outside consultants. Or the strategies may be developed less formally through interviews, facilitated sessions, or management retreats.

Regardless of the method used to define strategies, it is important that they are supported by executive management and that they are flexible. As the industry changes, the business strategies of any organization need to be continually revisited and updated. By definition then, the IT vision developed from the business strategies will also need continued refining.

The strategies below have been organized into several categories that support the environment defined by the industry

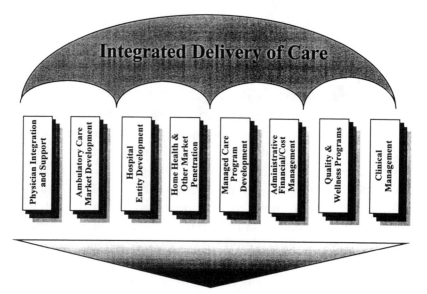

* Examples Only

Figure 2.4   *Your Enterprise . . . Business Strategies (Examples Only)*

trends and directions—an integrated delivery-of-care model based on capitation and integration of various providers, payers, and employers.

- *Physician Integration and Support.* Various types of provider groups are continually being formed; each has specific arrangements with the group members as well as with the organizations they support. The rapid development of these groups is in part a response to the consolidation of buying power in the health care industry. Primary care networks are very common; they provide gatekeeping functions for hospitals and managed care organizations as well as feeder functions to specialist groups. Health care organizations realize the foundation of much of their business revolves around successful relationships with the physician networks and view these groups as integral to the definition of business strategies.

- *Ambulatory-Care Market Development.* In an attempt to lower the costs of delivering health care, the industry has moved the setting of providing care away from the very expensive inpatient, acute-care environment. Primary-care centers, diagnostic laboratories, outpatient surgical centers, and other such facilities have emerged as key providers of care and are important in the business strategies of any health care organization. Additionally, as insurers include this type of care in reimbursement schemes and purchasers of health care demand these services in coverage, the health care organizations must include them in the strategic planning of the integrated delivery-of-care model.

- *Hospital Entity Development.* Although the hospital has changed from being viewed as the key to revenue generation and the center of care to a high-cost and, at times, less comforting solution (to the patient), the hospital unit is and will continue to be (at least in the near future) a key player in the integrated delivery-of-care model. The definition of what services are provided by this hospital and how the services are delivered will change rapidly, however. Integration of the hospital with the other components of the delivery-of-care model will be essential in providing low-cost, improved-quality, and customer-focused care in the future.

- *Home Health and Other Market Penetration.* Very much related to the ambulatory-care strategy, this strategy also focuses on developing lower-cost and improved-quality ways in which to deliver health care. In order to provide services along the full continuum of care, strategic business focus will be placed in care of patients before, during, and after treatment in inpatient setting. Examples include subacute care, hospice care, and nursing and long-term care facilities. Further, as hospital stays become shorter and care is moved out of the hospital, patients need attention at home during the recovery or maintenance periods.

- *Managed Care Program Development.* Depending on the part of the country and the stage of development of managed care, this strategy can be the most important in the organization's planning. Each facility will define this strategy in a different way, depending on how much risk the organization is willing to assume, on the legal and operational relationships with other providers, insurers, and even employers, and on many other factors. Organizations may choose to contract for managed care through a health maintenance organization (HMO) or a preferred provider organization (PPO), may have their own HMO, or may create other business arrangements.

- *Administrative and Financial Cost Management.* This strategy refers to the necessary infrastructure required to run the organization and consists of components such as patient accounting management, general and cost accounting, and other decision and support services. As the enterprisewide organizational structure develops, these administrative and financial strategies are essential to support the overall organization as well as each entity. Specific strategies in this area include development of a centralized business office, development of a management services organization, and potential outsourcing arrangements.

■ *Quality and Wellness Programs.* The recent attention on providing quality services has given rise to outcomes management, clinical protocols, and quality indicators. Integrated health care organizations want to be able to measure how care is delivered and therefore need consistent and statistically significant amounts of data related to the full treatment of care. Wellness programs aim to keep patients out of the hospital: Definitions of health status and high-risk patients are needed to help develop and achieve this strategy. Further, organizations are developing services to target high-risk activities such as smoking, drug abuse, and so on.

■ *Clinical Management.* This strategy includes the ability to manage each patient case from the perspective of different health providers (each with its own objectives). Case management must be integrated not only for the different providers involved in the case, but also over the continuum of care which will potentially occur in different inpatient and outpatient settings.

The Enterprise Information Technology Vision

In the previous sections, we presented an organized approach that will support the development of a tailored information technology vision by reviewing concepts and examples. This vision will ultimately be used during information systems planning to help rank and justify information technology projects.

After understanding the trends that affect the industry and information technology, and creating a well-supported definition of your enterprise's business strategies, you can proceed to the next step of strategic information technology planning: that of the *information technology vision* definition. Figure 2.5 shows a straw-man vision of a health-care enterprise. We will use this in the remainder of this chapter to help explain the components that need to be considered in the information technology visioning process.

We have divided the vision into three sections that will help define tools, techniques, and applications.

- *Enterprisewide or Common Section.* These tools, techniques, and applications are used across the enterprise. They may be shared by, for example, the hospital, ambulatory-care center, and the home health entity. Since the integrated delivery system vertically integrates the services provided to any one patient or member, these technologies allow utilization of different services in an efficient manner.

- *Entity-Specific Section.* These tools, techniques, and applications are specific to individual entities in the enterprise. For example, a system that provides functionality to an imaging center is not necessarily needed in a physician's office. As health care market factors and process reengineering changes the way health care is delivered, more entity-specific technologies will become enterprisewide. This migration will further streamline the processes and provide a more integrated way to treat patients and members.

- *Technical Section.* These enabling technologies provide the technical infrastructure that will allow and support the implementation of enterprisewide and

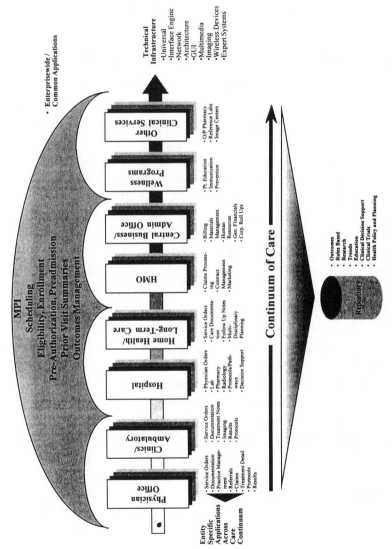

Figure 2.5 *Your Enterprise . . . Information Technology Vision*

35

entity-specific tools, techniques, and applications. Much of the technology has been deployed in other industries and has enabled those industries to provide more effective and user-oriented tools that enable competitive advantages needed in business.

Enterprisewide or Common Applications

As the health care industry continues to integrate horizontally, and as health care organizations provide services that span the continuum of care, applications to support this seamless integration must be procured or developed on the enterprisewide level. For example, a global registration and scheduling system provides a means to input and access patient or member demographic, clinical, and financial data. Generally this type of application is also integrated to a master person (patient or member) index. Each time the patient or member visits one of the entities, whether this is the hospital, surgery center, or outpatient pharmacy, the provider can access and update the most current information and not have to register the individual again.

Traditional and emerging *insurance applications* are also typical enterprisewide applications because the information provided in these systems is needed by virtually each entity in the integrated delivery system. Specifically, a hospital, subacute facility, or emergency-care center will each need to access eligibility and enrollment information as members present for treatment. Any preauthorizations or referrals need to be understood as early in the treatment process as possible to ensure appropriate reimbursement for services rendered.

Data repositories that contain patient, member, or guarantor information generated from all encounters with the enterprise are essential as health care organizations develop into businesses focused on the continuum of care. These repositories not only contain financial and administrative data, but they are also being defined to contain clinical data that will support outcomes management, clinical guidelines, and clinical decision-support applications. The repositories also need to collect (once the organization carefully defines) the most appropriate measures of quality, considering such factors as governing body standards (Joint Commission for Accreditation of Health Care Organizations and National Committee for Quality Assurance) and other mandates from employers and payers in the enterprise environment.

As discussed in the previous section, your enterprise should not skip immediately to the enterprisewide information technology vision without taking a very close look at the *operational processes* in place at the enterprise and entity-specific levels. It is essential to reengineer processes that were in place to support separately functioning businesses so that new processes, operations, and technology support an integrated delivery system.

Entity-Specific Applications

There are many types of entities in an integrated delivery system. Each operates with business strategies that relate to its core business as well as strategies that support the overall enterprise goals and objectives. This section reviews some of these entities and the information system tools, techniques, and applications associated with each type of operation. As the health care organization becomes more integrated and focused on clinical information processing, the particular systems requirements in each entity will overlap to an even greater degree, thus moving entity-specific applications into the category of enterprisewide technology support.

■ *Physician Offices and Businesses.* The information technology implications associated with this entity depend on the specific relationship each physician group has with the integrated delivery system. For example, group practices may be hospital based or independent. The groups may want anything from management support to total ownership management from the health care organization. Or the physicians may have a varied relationship with the organization, depending on the entity in the overall enterprise with which it is interacting (e.g., relationships of physicians in academic or university-based enterprises and their roles in treating clinic versus hospital-based patients).

Some specific information enabling-technology implications for these arrangements include ability to interface with the hospital systems; orders, lab results, and documentation functionality; claims processing and management; eligibility and enrollment capabilities; treatment detail, protocols, and clinical outcomes management.

■ *Clinics and Ambulatory Businesses.* As with physicians' offices, the enabling-technology implications in this environment vary depending on the entity's specific lines of business and strategies. Nevertheless, these facilities, often in remote locations (relative to the main inpatient facility), require access to the patient record from a clinical, demographic, and financial perspective. Caregivers want the ability to process orders, results, and documentation and treatment notes on-line as well as the ability to access historical information relevant to the patient.

■ The ability to transmit data, text, images, and audio from one remote facility to perhaps a larger facility staffed with specialists allows patient care to be delivered in lower-cost settings (avoiding transfers to inpatient facilities) as well as in settings more pleasing to the patients.

■ *Hospital Environments.* Enabling technologies in the inpatient environment are rapidly changing. Caregivers and administrators in the hospital environment need access to integrated patient information, whether it is from an on- or off-site ancillary department (radiology, physical therapy, etc.), ambulatory entities (e.g., surgery centers), or from the latest home health encounters. Management from the enterprise, in addition to hospital management desires tools to access executive information for decision support, and wants the ability to drill down into areas of concern for detailed information that reflects clinical and financial management of patients and members.

■ *Home Health and Long-Term Care.* Businesses such as these are often included in the integrated delivery system and have associated information system implications that depend on extensive integration and data repository support of different enterprise information systems. Specifically, the caregivers need access to all patient information that has been collected over the patient's stay(s) for inpatient and ambulatory services. This information helps assess and determine the additional treatment required and ensures the continuity of care in a quality manner. Specific application support includes service orders, care documentation, follow-up notes, miscellaneous patient-care planning, and durable medical equipment functionality.

■ *Health Maintenance Organizations.* As with the physician-oriented businesses, managed care arrangements such as HMOs, PPOs, and other payer ventures or arrangements may take on many business relationships with the enterprise. If there is a tight relationship between the enterprise and the managed care entity, and the enterprise has its own HMO, the system requirements may be significant: Application needs could range from enrollment or eligibility functions to claims processing and contract management capabilities, and even to clinical treatment protocols and measurements.

As the vision is developed in this area, it is important to consider how the enterprise wants to use information from this and other areas to gain a competitive advantage, especially over other providers who offer managed care products.

If there is a looser arrangement between the provider enterprise and the managed care entity, enterprise information application requirements could include sophisticated connection capabilities to allow data to be moved from one environment to another.

■ *Central Business Office and Administrative Offices.* Information systems implications in these areas depend on the organization structure of such administrative responsibilities. A centralized business office (CBO), for example, would require sophisticated information systems support, especially if the CBO supports different types of entities outside of the traditional acute-care inpatient environment. Other entity-specific applications include materials management, human resources, general accounting, and cost accounting.

As the enterprise becomes more integrated, information systems tools and support in this area will migrate into the section discussed above that contains enterprisewide or common technologies. For example, many integrated delivery systems are realizing more cost savings and operational efficiencies by consolidating materials management and purchasing functions of the various entities; thus the information systems would also need to be consolidated. Through the visioning process, the review of such issues is essential to ensure that the vision and the resulting information systems plans are supportive of the future migration of the enterprise.

■ *Wellness Programs.* Such programs include patient education, immunization, and prevention. Information needs in this area include specific encounter information, patient or member health profiles, and clinical trends that help the enterprise determine new opportunities for services. Clinical data from various sources are required as well as comparative data on treatment alternatives. Lastly, other requirements may include predictive data on costs to maintain the health of the patients and members in the enterprise community.

■ *Clinical Services.* These services include outpatient pharmacies, reference labs, and radiology centers. Each service has unique information requirements, yet the overall information vision for future needs is similar to the above entities: These businesses require access to updated patient information from all sources that treated or interacted with the individual. This type of information is critical to help deliver quality care in the most effective and patient-focused way possible.

Technical Infrastructure

The technical infrastructure in the overall information technology visioning exercise is a critical consideration. Without including these technologies in the visioning exercise, the ultimate information systems planning and design will be limited, and the chances of being able to build upon existing architectures and applications as the environment changes will be significantly decreased.

As discussed in the section on information systems trends and technologies, tools such as universal interface engines, graphical user interfaces, telemedicine, imaging, wireless technology, and expert systems will not only improve information processing, but will also allow users the flexibility to improve business processes. Additionally, emerging technologies considered in the visioning exercise will provide framework for developing a truly seamless view of patient and member information across the enterprise.

Summary: Where to Now?

The enterprise's information technology vision provides a strategic link between the critical business strategies and goals of an enterprise, the business processes that enable those strategies, and the technologies that support the processes. As we have shown, influences of the ultimate information technology vision for each enterprise include trends and directions from the health care industry and information technology, as well as the specific enterprise strategies and process models.

Investments in information technology to support integrated delivery systems will continue to be significant. The risks associated with these investments can be minimized through the development of an informational technology vision along with a strategic and tactical implementation plan. Paying attention to external business and technology factors as well as understanding the direction of your organization, are essential elements in the visioning process. Equally important is the attention given to understanding current processes in your organization and the ways in which these processes can be streamlined. Reengineered processes function in a symbiotic action with information technology to ultimately allow investments in such technology to support and enable the strategies and goals of your enterprise.

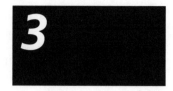

3

Reengineering the Process

Overview

Having developed an information technology vision for the health care organization, administrators are faced with the task of developing an IT strategy that will bridge the current state to the future-state vision. Developing this bridging strategy is a complex process incorporating elements of current processes, existing IT capabilities, and the ability of vendors in the marketplace to support new requirements. It is essential that the strategic planning effort validate existing and reengineered processes as well as vendor capabilities in order to deliver a viable and comprehensive solution. This validation process reduces the risk associated with inflated expectations and market hype about technologies that may seem promising but do not necessarily align with the organization's strategic goals and objectives.

Understanding existing processes and how they are being redefined to cross functional lines is critical for assessing the role of information technology as an enabler of change. Many technologies available today have been developed under a fee-for-service paradigm supporting processes that are now changing along with the industry. The result is that new demands are being placed on information systems, and new challenges are forcing organizations to search for different strategies to manage care and compete effectively.

Reengineering existing processes is a multistep effort that often affects departments normally considered out of scope for a particular function. The effort involves building a business case, documenting existing processes with cycle times and volumes, identifying opportunities for improvement, conducting cost/benefit analyses, and developing the new process. The new "future state" process reflects the organization's vision as well as realities of existing conditions and ability to implement change.

The Case for Change

Building a business case to motivate change is an often under-emphasized element of many projects. Lack of a clear business case is one of the most pronounced reasons many strategic plans collect dust on the executive bookshelf. The business case provides the motivational component required to gain consensus and implement change. Building the business case requires analysis of a number of factors, including local penetration of managed care, employer initiatives, and competition. While specific conditions cannot be addressed in a text such as this, observations can be made on national trends and market conditions.

The most consequential trend today in the health care industry is in the way employers are purchasing health care. Skyrocketing health care costs are forcing employers to undertake aggressive cost-containment efforts. The result is a movement toward managed care plans that are proving to be more effective in controlling health care costs. Figure 3.1 shows the advantage managed care plans are demonstrating over traditional indemnity plans for large employer groups. Figure 3.2 shows that managed care for small employers is also becoming a cost-effective alternative to traditional indemnity plans.

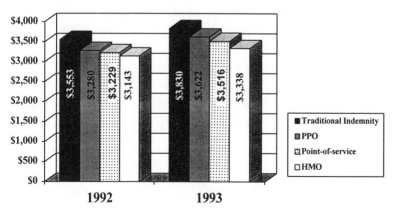

Figure 3.1   *Health Plan Costs for Large Employers*

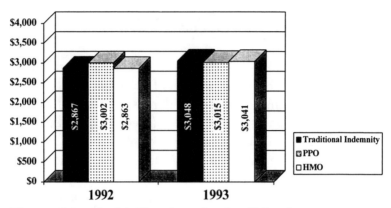

Figure 3.2   *Health Plan Costs for Small Employers*

Additionally, the Group Health Association of America (GHAA) reported that in 1995 the average HMO member premium dropped by 1.2 percent. This drop in premiums is dramatic in an industry that has grown accustomed to a very high rate of inflation over the last decade. This dramatic reversal is due to the competitive nature of managed care organizations and their effectiveness in controlling health care costs.

This effectiveness cannot be matched by indemnity plans. In fact, as managed care plans become more cost-effective, indemnity plans get caught in what is called a "death spiral." The death spiral is a situation where indemnity plans become increasingly more expensive every year as healthier members flee to managed care plans, and higher utilizers continue to sign with the indemnity plan.

A growing number of employers are recognizing the difference between managed care plans and indemnity plans, and these employers are taking action. According to a Foster-Higgins Employee Benefits Services study of 979 mid-sized employers:

■   The number of mid-sized employers offering traditional indemnity plans declined from 61 percent in 1992 to 57 percent in 1993.

■   Nearly 24 percent of mid-sized employers offered a PPO in 1993, up from 21 percent in 1992.

■ The use of point-of-service (POS) plans among mid-sized employers doubled in 1993, from 2 percent in 1992 to 4 percent in 1993.

■ Of these employers, 21 percent offered an HMO; this number remained steady through 1993.

These trends also point toward another major shift in the health care industry—health care organizations are realizing they must now view the purchaser of health care (government, employer, or consumer) as the customer. Health plans succeed in this business climate by focusing on cost, quality, and access. Cost competitiveness and access are required to gain membership and quality is required to retain that membership. Providers succeed in this business climate by solidifying per-member, per-month revenue streams. This is done by catering to the needs of health plans and also focusing on the same customer service objectives of cost, quality, and access.

Document Existing Processes

The first step in reengineering a process is to document the existing process in a series of process-flow diagrams. The current process flow serves as the baseline for conducting cost/benefit analysis, assessing the scope of change, and implementation planning. The level of detail required depends on the complexity of the process and detail expected by executive management for them to accept the analyses and approve organizational changes.

The baseline process flow should document the following types of information:

■ Individual tasks at the individual job function level

■ Volumes for each activity (e.g., occurrences per day, month, or year)

■ Cycle times for each activity

- Staffing levels for each function

- Wait times

- Handoffs

- Rework and other nonvalue-added activities

- Authorization activities

- Use of technology or other tools

Before conducting the data collection effort it is prudent to understand exactly what information you need and how you will use the information. Data-collection efforts without clear direction usually end up wasting time and frustrating project participants. Frequently, simply documenting existing processes leads to quick-hit improvement initiatives that become self-evident once the process is profiled and analyzed.

Identifying Opportunities for Improvement

The health care industry is changing the way processes are viewed. Under fee for service, processes are viewed at a departmental level: lab, pharmacy, radiology, emergency department, registration, intensive care, operating room, and so on, due to the reimbursement schedule. The reimbursement structure encourages separation between departments, leaving little incentive for collaboration. Managed care, on the other hand, is blind to departmental boundaries and rewards overall efficiencies. Managed care, therefore, rewards collaboration between departments or facilities and supports a comprehensive view of the health care process. The comprehensive view of the process is forcing health care organizations to rethink how they invest in technology.

In this new environment, information technology must be able to demonstrate value, and the value must measure beyond the bounds of departmental-level processes. Tom Davenport, in *Process Innovation: Reengineering Work through Information Technology,* advocates the importance of measuring the value of information technology outside the boundaries of current processes: "If nothing changes about the way work is done and the role of IT is simply to automate an existing process, economic benefits are likely to be minimal."

This perspective of the process enables administrators to escape the traditional departmental boundaries and search for improvement opportunities along the entire continuum of care. The results can be impressive. For example, a recent study illustrated the potential of simply making information readily accessible to physicians. Health science librarians at the Medical Library Association studied the effect of on-line literature-searching on the length of stay and patient care costs in three Michigan hospitals. The study showed that a statistically significant relationship exists between the use of information from searching databases for severely ill patients and reductions in their lengths of stay and hospital costs. According to the study, conducting literature searches earlier in patient hospital stays reduces costs by 70 percent, charges billed to the patients by 68 percent, and lengths of stay by 65 percent.

This simple example illustrates the value of looking beyond departmental boundaries. In this case the added effort by librarians in assisting physicians resulted in a dramatic reduction in overall costs. Examples like this are compelling and provide a measure by which the value of easy access to information can be measured.

The change in the way processes are viewed is also changing the way technology is employed. In the past, individual departments often were given autonomy to select information systems based on their departmental needs. These systems provide minimal value to areas outside the department and, as has also been shown, do not always provide value within the department, either. Additionally, this type of flexibility in decentralized system selection results in headaches for CIOs who are inevitably asked to integrate them into the existing environment.

Competition in the marketplace is forcing many administrators to rethink this approach. Budgets are even tighter than before, and departmental autonomy in selecting systems is not an effective way to maximize available resources. In no way can technology be applied in an innovative way when it is selected based on a narrowly defined needs profile. Michael Hammer and James Champy, in *Reengineering the Corporation: A Manifesto for Business Revolution,* summarize the error in looking at technology with limited goals.

> The fundamental error that most companies commit when they look at technology is to view it through the lens of their existing processes. They ask, "How can we use these new technological capabilities to enhance or streamline or improve what we are already doing?" Instead, they should be asking, "How can we use technology to allow us to do things that we are *not* already doing?"

As identified by Hammer and Champy, part of the value of information technology can only be measured in its ability to support unforeseen demands. The measure is in its flexibility. In today's dynamic health care environment, flexibility cannot be underemphasized. Tom Peters stresses this point in his own summary of his best-selling management book: "The chief axiom of *Thriving on Chaos* is the necessity of attaining, and then maintaining, heretofore undreamed-of flexibility."

The emergence of horizontally and vertically integrated delivery systems is the principle result of increased competition in the health care industry. Integrated delivery systems offer the most potential for controlling costs because incentive structures are aligned, and there is new opportunity to reengineer the complete health care process. These advantages become more evident when integrated delivery systems are compared to regular HMOs. Figure 3.3 and Figure 3.4 illustrate the advantages integrated delivery systems are experiencing over traditional HMOs.

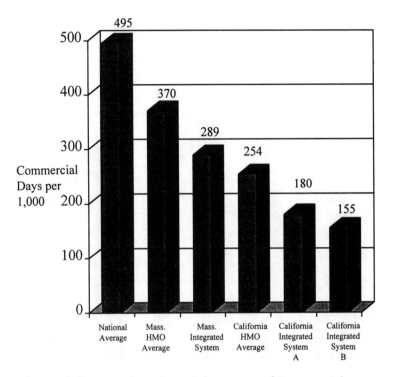

Figure 3.3 *Inpatient Days Advantage of Integrated Delivery Systems*

Much of the advantage integrated delivery systems have shown thus far is due to the complete alignment of incentives throughout the enterprise. However, integrated delivery systems are not resting on their laurels as they are beginning to take advantage of information technology to support comprehensive reengineering efforts. Integrated delivery systems are discovering newfound opportunities for realizing value through information technology.

Understanding the potential benefits of a well-integrated delivery system, the next question is how to begin reengineering a process to achieve an advantage. Many integrated systems consist of hospitals, physicians, and other health care organizations that are not comfortable working together and rely on a

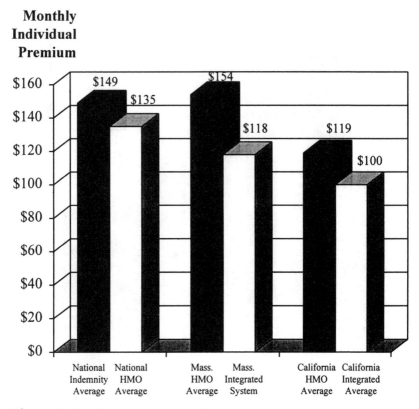

Figure 3.4   *Cost Advantage of Integrated Delivery Systems*

variety of disparate technologies for administrative and clinical support.

One approach to process reengineering relies on the use of value propositions and developing a portfolio of improvement initiatives. Figure 3.5 illustrates the process of developing an improvement portfolio. The process starts with the identification of value propositions. Value propositions are ideas for improving the existing process. They may utilize technology or they may simply involve elimination of nonvalue-added activities.

Value propositions can best be illustrated by looking at a situation many large health systems encounter as they attempt to streamline operations and leverage resources across an

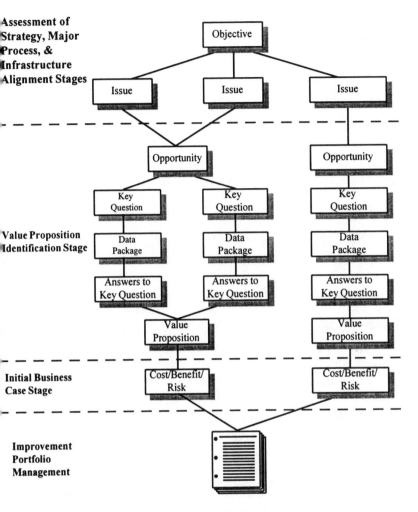

Figure 3.5 *Improvement Portfolio Development*

expanding enterprise. The radiology function, for example, is an area where large health systems may realize efficiencies and improve customer service by optimizing resources across many previously independent radiology departments. In this case, the mega-process is radiology, and the scope includes pre-admission planning to discharge and spans multiple episodes of care. The radiology mega process can be broken into nine subprocesses.

1. Radiology Order Generation

2. Radiology Procedure Scheduling

3. Transportation

4. Examinations/Procedures

5. Reading/Interpretation/Dictation

6. Report Transcription/Validation/Production

7. Film Storage/Archive/Retrieval

8. Billing

9. Executive Reporting

Value propositions are developed against these subprocesses. Value propositions may apply to a single subprocess or may span several subprocesses. Additionally, the initial list of value propositions may include contradicting proposals. Contradictions will we worked out later when the propositions are rank ordered and the new processes are engineered. Value propositions may employ sophisticated equipment or may be as simple as improved training. Different value propositions will support different objectives.

Examples of value propositions for a multifacility radiology department might include:

1. Radiology Order Generation—Value Propositions
   - Build exam protocols into critical pathways and clinical guidelines
   - Automatically schedule exams upon admission based on diagnosis or procedure
   - Support order placement in a manner that smooths demand for radiology resources
   - Eliminate duplicate or contradictory orders via auto verification and use of systems edits

- Automate order entry/verification/authorization process

2. Radiology Procedure Scheduling—Value Propositions
   - Centralize patient scheduling function to support more effective allocation of resources
   - Schedule patient at site convenient for the patient
   - Load patient demographic/clinical information in the radiology system prior to exam via interface engine
   - Employ a system to support more efficient scheduling of radiology staff
   - Ensure appropriate staffing levels for weekends and holidays; also ensure proper coverage during breaks and shift changes

3. Transportation—Value Propositions
   - Redeploy selected radiology equipment closer to patient-care units
   - Employ portable radiology equipment
   - Employ teleradiology to reduce patient transport and reduce film walking
   - Reduce dead-end/duplicate transportation runs
   - Centralize radiology equipment to a single location (applies to health systems made up of several hospitals or other facilities)

4. Examinations/Procedures—Value Propositions
   - Incorporate exam/procedure protocols in critical paths
   - Enhance or refine existing procedure protocols
   - Reduce film developing and handling costs through bulk purchasing or outsourcing

5. Reading/Interpretation/Dictation—Value Propositions
   - Automatically retrieve clinically relevant films from previous exams
   - Provide access to knowledge base of previous exams

- Centralize radiology readings
- Provide remote reading service for clinics, physician offices, affiliates, and outreach services
- Employ voice recognition technology for report generation
- Employ mouse driven or touch screen technology to enable radiologists to compile reports by selecting canned phrases
- Employ transcriptionist to take real-time face-to-face dictation
- Employ transcriptionist to take real-time dictation using groupware application (the transcriptionist would stay in the transcription pool)
- Utilize standard (canned) reports for simple, high volume exams such as mammography

6. Report Transcription/Validation/Production—Value Propositions
   - Centralize transcription service
   - Real-time dictation/transcription
   - Eliminate preliminary report running
   - Provide on-line access to report for validation
   - Implement automatic signature for medical record copy
   - Make recorded dictation available to attending physicians as soon as dictation is complete

7. Film Storage/Archive/Retrieval—Value Propositions
   - Enhance film access and tracking system
   - Support keyword searches of selected reports for research purposes
   - Reduce manual film retrievals to only clinically relevant films
   - Implement a picture archiving and communication systems (PACS)
   - Provide standard resolution access to images via bedside terminals

8. Billing—Value Propositions
   - Improve charge capture and patient billing procedures
   - Calibrate costing method for improved tracking
   - Enhance utilization tracking and reporting for managed care contracts

9. Executive Reporting—Value Propositions
   - Provide better access to utilization and financial statistics

After an initial set of value propositions has been identified, the next step is to assess the costs and benefits of each proposition and to build the future state processes. While value propositions may seem generic, the manner in which they are prioritized and implemented will vary considerably. Specific market conditions and overall direction and vision of the organization will greatly influence how the reengineered future state process operates.

In today's market, the local penetration of managed care and the organization's perception of managed care is the largest single factor influencing process reengineering. Aligned goals under a managed care system support the implementation of new technologies that have hard-to-measure value under a fee-for-service paradigm. An example of this type of technology is a computer-based patient record (CPR) system, which is designed to facilitate easy access to clinical information and support direct entry of information by the physician or other caregiver (see Chapter 6). Computer-based patient record systems also hold the key to measuring outcomes and supporting better patient flow across the continuum of care—critical elements of a well-managed health care system.

Under a fee-for-service paradigm, a CPR system must demonstrate value to each of the individual stakeholders in order to be fully accepted. A major obstacle is in acceptance and use by physicians. CPR systems can provide value in a number of areas, but they have not been able to demonstrate an ability to enable physicians to increase productivity. In fact, during the implementation of a CPR, physicians will endure a learning curve, and productivity will likely suffer. After the learning curve is over, volumes reach historical levels but likely will not exceed them. To a physician receiving reimbursement under a fee-for-service structure, this translates into reduced income in the worst case and increased hassle in the best case. In essence, the fee-for-service reimbursement structure discourages acceptance of the technology.

Under a capitated structure or other structure where rewards are based on the efficiency of the entire system (managed care), physicians do not need to be cajoled into using a CPR system. Physicians who have an equity position or are recipients of risk pool payouts may better understand that their income is tied to more than just personal productivity. Therefore they have an incentive to use the system.

Similar fee-for-service or managed care analogies can be applied to other technologies such as clinical guidelines, health information networks, and telemedicine. The reasons for choosing a technology are no longer to satisfy the needs of an individual department or functional area but those of the entire health system. Accordingly, the criteria for selecting a technology are different and the processes that must be supported are more encompassing.

Building the Future State Process

Integrated delivery systems have an advantage in their ability to address the entire process when applying technology and identifying reengineering opportunities. Reengineering the complete process has clearly proved advantageous in other industries. Ford Motor Company, for example, learned about the value of looking at the entire process when it was searching for ways to reduce head count in its bloated accounts payable (AP) department. In the early 1980s Ford believed it could reduce head count in its AP department of 500 employees by 20 percent. Ford had recently acquired a 25 percent equity interest in Mazda, and project planners decided to take a look at Mazda's AP department. Ford executives were surprised to find that Mazda supported the AP function with 5 people. The planners quickly realized that they had to rethink the role of AP within a larger process.

Ford ended up reengineering the more encompassing procurement process, setting up the process so shipments could be verified against purchase orders when they were received at the loading dock. Vendors were asked not to send invoices and, consequently, the task of matching invoices to purchase orders in AP was completely eliminated. Ford now has an AP department of 125, still more than Mazda, but significantly fewer than the original target of 400.

This solution combined a comprehensive view of the process with enabling technologies to produce quantum improvements in the way products and services were delivered. Reengineering publications are filled with similar examples of enormous improvements through innovative uses of information technology.

As health care is transformed into a cost-competitive industry, there will be similar innovative applications of information technology. Furthermore, health care will soon join ranks of other industries that depend on information technology for survival. Technology will soon enable new processes in medical management, clinical pathways, and product development. Michael Hammer and James Champy, in *Reengineering the Corporation,* discuss the effect of technology on corporations in general:

> Technology changes the nature of competition in ways companies don't expect. In retailing, for instance, it has allowed manufacturers and retailers, such as Procter & Gamble and Wal-Mart, to merge their distribution and inventory systems in the ways that are mutually beneficial.

It is likely that technology will change health care in ways that most organizations will not expect. One area that is likely to see a significant transformation is the development of clinical guidelines and critical pathways. Currently many health care organizations are in the process of developing clinical guidelines and critical pathways, and they are already experiencing significant gains. These efforts focus on defining a guideline or path based on consensus among physicians. However, they have yet to incorporate comprehensive outcome measures, enabled by IT. They also have yet to consider the potential of information technology to streamline the care delivery process. This is mostly due to the lack of mature technologies supporting this area and the overall inexperience of physicians in using computers. In the future, however, this will change as technology becomes more pervasive in health care. The first organizations that successfully build clinical pathways around enabling technologies will gain a significant competitive advantage in the marketplace.

Measure the Process

In classic Total Quality Management (TQM), measurement is the key for improving the process. "Measurement is the heart of any improvement process. If something cannot be measured, it cannot be improved," says Jim Harrington, senior Ernst & Young quality manager and 1986 chairman of the American Society for Quality Control. In the West, the four best-known quality management experts are Philip Crosby, the late W. Edwards Deming, Armand V. Feigenbaum, and Joseph Juran. Each of these experts has a distinct approach to quality management, but one of the common themes is the importance of measuring. The ability to measure results is an essential element of process improvement. Accordingly, information technology must support this measurement process.

In health care, measuring outcomes is becoming increasingly important as health care providers search for ways to reduce costs and attract patients. Measuring outcomes is crucial to reducing length of stays, utilization, and unnecessary procedures. Under fee for service and even prospective payment systems such as Medicare, there is little incentive to reduce unnecessary procedures; in fact, the incentive is for more procedures. Under managed care, however, there is a clear incentive to reduce unnecessary procedures. Managed care administrators are only beginning to realize the potential in this area. One recent example that illustrates this point is in a study from Harvard Medical School, which concludes that 25 percent of invasive procedures performed on elderly heart attack victims—catheterizations, balloon angioplasties, and coronary bypasses—could be eliminated with no effect on patients' survival. The study team found that elderly heart attack victims had lower mortality rates in New York, where 15 percent were catheterized, than in California and Texas, where 27 percent underwent the procedure. The price tag for the unnecessary procedures, in this example, was $600 million.

Studies like this are conclusive and clearly illustrate the potential for savings if the correct incentive structures are put into place and necessary information is made readily available to caregivers. The unfortunate element of this example is that the study required a team of researchers to focus on one issue for an extended period of time. This example illustrates the need for information technology to enable processes that are not possible in a nonautomated or inflexible environment. With the right type of information systems, health plan administrators should be able to perform studies like this in 10 minutes. With this we can begin to see that the real value of information technology lies in the ability to support future, unplanned information needs and processes.

It is naive, however, to believe that we can easily adapt information that is structured for other purposes to meet new needs. This point was made clear by a study conducted by the

New England Health Plan Employer Data Information Set (HEDIS) Coalition in 1994. The Coalition evaluated the results of data provided by 15 health plans serving the region. (HEDIS asks for a set of 160 performance indicators in the areas of clinical quality, finances, member access and satisfaction, membership stability, and resource utilization.) One finding of the study was that a higher rate of preventive screening was measured by health plans that sampled medical records than by health plans that simply measured through existing administrative records. This discrepancy was not due to actual differences in screening rates, but rather to the source of the information used. In this case, use of existing information systems to measure outcomes led to an underreporting of performance. This disparity illustrates the potential value behind well-planned, flexible information technology that could support accurate outcomes measurement.

Summary

Under fee for service, information technology had to address and satisfy the needs of a diverse group of customers and a diverse set of processes. Consequently, it was extremely difficult to implement a technology that satisfies the requirements of all stakeholders. Under managed care the consumer or employer is the customer, and goals are aligned so that all stakeholders' needs and requirements ultimately map to the objectives of lower cost, higher quality, and better access. This alignment of goals changes the way value is measured and information systems are selected.

These changes are both a blessing and a curse for CIOs. It is a blessing because it will be easier to identify and measure the value technology will provide to the organization. It is a curse because the scope has increased significantly, and CIOs may be more accountable to the success or failure of technology that has been implemented. Additionally, selected technologies must map directly to the organization's future state-vision. That vision sets the stage for defining processes that must be supported and the types of relationships that affect selection and evaluation methodologies.

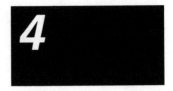

4

Assessing Your Strengths

Introduction

In today's health care market there are several reasons why an organization may choose to assess the current state of their information systems (IS), including:

Migrating to the Future-State Vision. A realistic assessment of the organization, application, and technical resources currently in place is needed to develop an implementation plan for the future-state vision (see Chapter 2: Developing a Vision). In addition, you need to understand your information services organization, including its skill set and its ability to support existing new technologies and applications.

Improving Current Operations. Even if your customers are well satisfied and the environment is relatively stable, organizations need to continually improve the effectiveness of their information technology function. This could involve reducing operating expenses, improving data security and privacy protocols, meeting compliance guidelines from Joint Commission for Accreditation of Health Care Organizations (JCAHO), or providing professional development opportunities for information services staff. These kinds of improvement opportunities will surface by conducting a current-state information technology assessment.

Effecting Mergers and Consolidations. Mergers, consolidations, and affiliations between health care organizations are continuing at a rapid pace. A critical component of the success of a merger can be the consolidation or integration of disparate sets of applications and technologies. In this example, analyzing the current state of the organization is critical when attempting to understand the resources (organization, application, and technology) that exist at each organization and develop a plan for consolidating the applications and technologies.

This chapter covers the basic elements of technology assessment and methods for collecting the information required to complete this analysis.

Information Gathering

Before discussing the components of an information technology assessment, let's discuss how to gather the information necessary to perform the analysis. There are several methods for gathering the information required to analyze the current environment, including questionnaires, one-on-one interviews, facilitated sessions, or more. Typically a combination of these is used. The information-gathering process involves discussions with senior executives, key users, and representatives from the information services department. The key objective of the information-gathering process is to obtain a comprehensive picture of the current state of information systems and how these systems support the current business strategy, critical success factors, and future vision of the organization.

Senior executive interviews provide an overall understanding of the organizational goals and key business strategies for the enterprise. Departmental or user interviews address the following points:

- Existing tactical plans for the department

- Current state of existing applications and technologies used within the department

- Future plans for the department

- Information systems objectives, functions, and reporting strategies

- Organizational structure and staffing levels within the department

■ User's satisfaction

■ User's understanding of the change-request process

These points are typically covered at two levels within the department—with senior and operational management. Senior management discussions focus on departmental business goals, current processes, future plans, and critical success factors. It is important to analyze these departmental goals against the organization's business strategy to fully understand the priority of projects both from a departmental and organizational perspective. A key responsibility of the information services department is to assist users with automation in their respective departments. Understanding user priorities and organizational priorities supports the process of setting information systems priorities.

The reviews at the operational level focus on the current state of existing applications and technology within the department and future information systems objectives. Applications supported by the information services department as well as other applications operating in the user departments (e.g., in-house-developed spreadsheets or databases for tracking or reporting, etc.) are included in this review. In addition, an understanding of the funding sources for new technologies (i.e., departmental budget or information services department budget) and the extent of departmental involvement in the selection, implementation, and maintenance processes is critical. This understanding provides input to the priority-setting process and is also important from an implementation planning perspective. Implementing new systems results in a level of change, and it is important that the information services department assists users in working through the change process. Therefore, understanding the relationship between the information services department and the user department can support the implementation planning process.

Interviews with representatives of the information services department cover the basics of how the information services department functions. Typically the interviews are conducted with the chief information officer, director, project leaders, select programming staff, and select operations support individuals. Specific points include assessing:

- Organizational structure of the department

- Current application and technology projects in process

- Projects planned for the future

- IS effectiveness and relationship with user departments

- Support processes for new and existing technologies

- Information technology capital and operating budgets

- IS staffing levels, mix, and skill sets

- Makeup, function, and effectiveness of IS user committees or steering committees

- Project prioritization, assignment, and tracking

- Standards for project reporting

- Data security and confidentiality

The result of the IS interviews is a thorough understanding of the organizational structure of the information services department. This includes how information technology standards and principles are deployed, what applications and technologies are currently in place, what staff is assigned to support these technologies, what level of documentation of current applications and projects exists, and what project support, tracking, planning, and reporting methodologies are used by the organization.

The result of the information-gathering process is an understanding of the relationship between the information services department and the organization as a whole: how information system projects are established in relation to organizational priorities, how timeliness of projects is developed and approved, what the relationship is between information services and the user departments, and what the organizational support for information systems is in terms of budgeted dollars.

Components of the Current State Assessment

To gain a full understanding of the true current state of the information systems within an entity, it is important to evaluate the organizational, application, and technology architectures that are in place as shown in Figure 4.1.

An organizational assessment entails evaluating all resources (people and dollars) that support information systems applications and technologies. As part of the organizational assessment, it is critical to develop an understanding of how the organization adapts to change as well as how the organization manages the change process. New technology implementations and organizational consolidations represent a significant change to any enterprise.

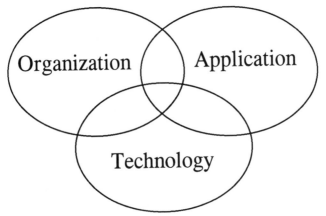

Figure 4.1   *Strategic Information Systems Plan Architectures*

An application assessment covers all applications in production as well as all application projects in process or being planned for the future. Many health care organizations support multiple lines of business (acute care, rehabilitation, long-term care, etc.), and it is imperative to gain an understanding of the applications currently supporting these businesses as well as the requirements for future applications and technologies.

A technology assessment includes an analysis of all platforms that support existing applications and any projects in progress to introduce new technologies. In many cases, organizations operate several technology platforms that support the traditional accounting and transaction-based systems. The technology assessment involves evaluating not only the platforms required to support these applications but also the skill sets and integration strategies in place to support connectivity between the platforms.

There are many aspects of each component that need to be evaluated. Each component and its associated steps will be discussed in more detail in the remainder of the chapter.

Organizational Assessment

Since the purpose of the organizational assessment is to focus on the resources throughout the entity dedicated to the support of information systems, it is important to note that IS resources can be internal to the information services department or external because they may reside in user departments. Information systems resource location, responsibility, and budget dollars (costs) are identified in the information-gathering process. To gain a full understanding of all resources available to support new applications and technologies, it is important to identify and assess all IS resources throughout the organization.

Information related to the information services department organization is typically summarized according to the following categories:

- Information services department structure

- Information services operations

- Information services principles and standards

- Information services budget

This depicts the level of resources required to support the existing applications and technology for the current state. Each of these is discussed in greater detail below.

Information Services Department Structure

The organization infrastructure for IS needs to support the changing functional needs of user departments. The organization structure needs to be flexible enough to support maintenance of existing systems concurrently with implementation of new technologies. In order to not fragment the department, it is important that the IS infrastructure be supported by staff with strong communication and project planning skills.

Figure 4.2 depicts a sample IS organizational chart at the functional level for a single entity organization. The typical IS organization consists of a technical component with resources to support the daily operations and tuning of systems and networks. Application analysts support the implementation of systems and work with users to define systems needs. Many organizations that support multiple business units divide IS support by the business unit (financial systems, clinical systems, administrative systems, long-term care functions, etc.).

Other functional responsibilities sometimes found within the IS department include training and biomedical engineering. Training is a large segment of any systems implementation, and trainers need to work closely with IS resources and users to ensure all functions of new applications are included in the training plan. A second area that is increasingly being linked to IS is biomedical engineering. Some organizations have shifted the responsibility of biomedical engineering to the CIO because in many cases, the biomedical resources need to work together

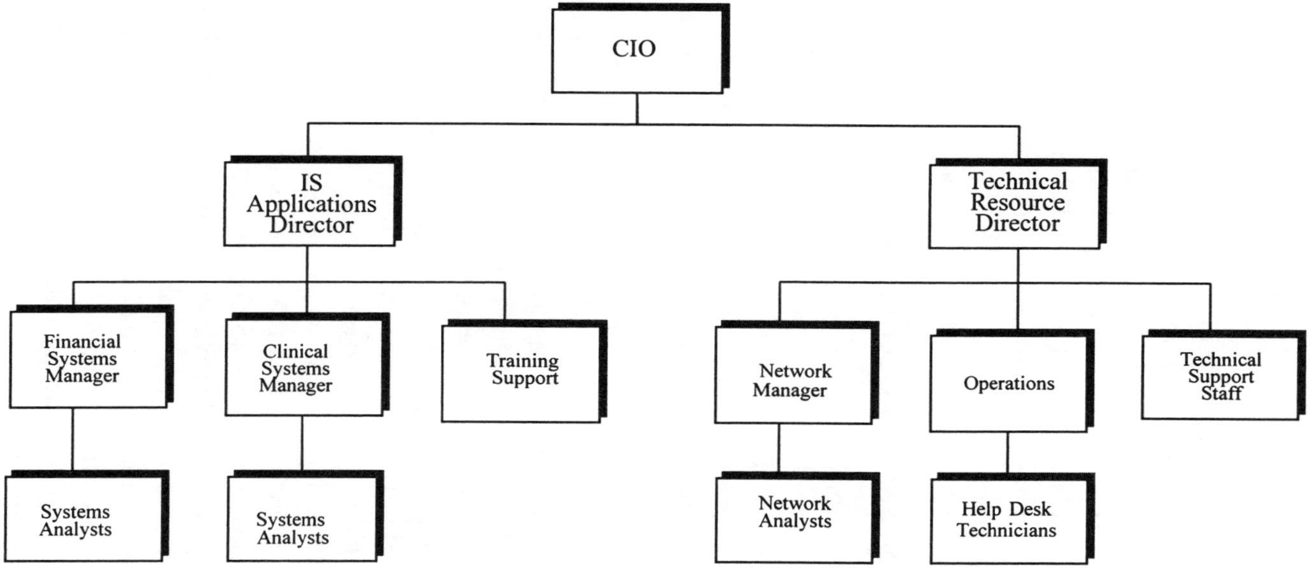

Figure 4.2 *Sample IS Organization Chart*

with the technical or network group to ensure integration of equipment with systems. Also the IS technical group and biomedical engineers often share a similar skill set (e.g., personal computer/technical maintenance and repair) which can be consolidated into one single group.

When evaluating the IS organizational structure, you should understand the culture and needs of the organization. No matter what the structure, it is critical that the IS analysts work closely with technical resources to understand user needs and develop integrated solutions that are feasible to implement. (See Chapter 7: The People Part for a discussion of IS organizations.)

Information Services Operations

During the information-gathering process, daily operation of systems, perceived level of support, and skill set of IS resources will be examined. It is important to understand the skill set and assignment of resources currently available within the IS department and the level of support applied to daily operation of existing applications.

When evaluating user satisfaction, you should evaluate all aspects, including daily support of applications, networks, PCs, and printers as well as implementation of new projects. A fine balance needs to be maintained between ongoing maintenance of daily operating systems and projects to implement new applications. Even if the majority of new applications are installed on time and within budget, users will still be frustrated and dissatisfied with IS support if, for example, the face sheet printers in the registration department are perceived to be always down.

Tools are available to streamline some of the daily operational functions within the IS department. Help desk software is available that supports tracking and follow-up of user calls for systems problems and application changes and updates. Lights Out operation applications are available to schedule running of daily, weekly, monthly, and periodic programs. Project management software is available to support project planning and tracking functions as well as resource allocation across all projects, including maintenance of current applications and new implementations.

Figure 4.3 shows a framework for categorizing skills by type of resources for existing applications, including those resources that may not directly report to IS.

The assessment of skill mix needs to take into consideration the skills that will be required to enhance existing applications and build the framework for new applications. The assessment should evaluate current skill sets of all IS resources with a focus on their ability to learn and support new applications and technologies.

As health care organizations move toward an integrated environment with wide area networks, computerized systems that use interface engines, and leading-edge technology, it will be important to acquire advanced knowledge of networking, interface standards, and specialized programming languages such as C++ and other rapid-application development tools.

An IS resource education plan is a critical component of the migration strategy to the future state. The education plan covers gaps in the IS department skills for supporting new technologies and shows the types of training that staff in the department will need to acquire. Another way to fill the gaps is to hire additional staff with the requisite skills.

Information Services Principles and Standards

It is becoming increasingly important for the information services department to position itself to support leading-edge technology and diverse organizational needs. In order to be successful, today's IS organization needs to be customer oriented with a focus on standards that support flexibility to quickly address systems issues, new regulations, and rapidly evolving technologies. These include:

- Standards for technology selection (application and hardware)
- Standard processes for requesting services

Current State: Skills Utilization

		Hardware	OS: UNIX	OS: Multiple	OS: Other	App. Support	Monitoring
Information Services:	Manager, IS	✓				✓	✓
	Operations Supervisor	✓				✓	✓
	Operations Support	✓			✓	✓	✓
	Phys. Acc. Netw. Tech.						
	PC Specialist						
	Programmer						
	Netw. Mgr./Specialist						
Clinical Engineering:	Director, Clinical Eng.	✓	✓		✓	✓	✓
	Assistant Director	✓	✓	✓	✓	✓	✓
	Sr. Biomed., Specialist	✓	✓		✓	✓	✓
	Cert. Biomed. Specialist	✓			✓		✓
	PC Service Specialist						✓
	Biomed, Equip. Tech.			✓		✓	
Cancer Center:	Research Coordinator						
Cost Accounting:	Accountant					✓	✓
Food & Nutrition:	System Coordinator						
Laboratory:	Informatics Manager	✓				✓	✓
	Computer Operator	✓				✓	✓
Materials Mgmt:	System Coordinator					✓	
Medical Records:	Supervisor Transcription	✓				✓	
	Coding Specialists					✓	
Nursing:	System Coordinator						
Pharmacy:	Supervisors					✓	
Quality Assurance:	Supervisor						
Radiology:	System Coordinator	✓				✓	

Figure 4.3   *Current State: Skills Utilization*

- ■ Standard approaches to reporting problems

- ■ A methodology for managing projects with a project team concept

- ■ Standards for accomplishing various activities (such as PC hardware installation)

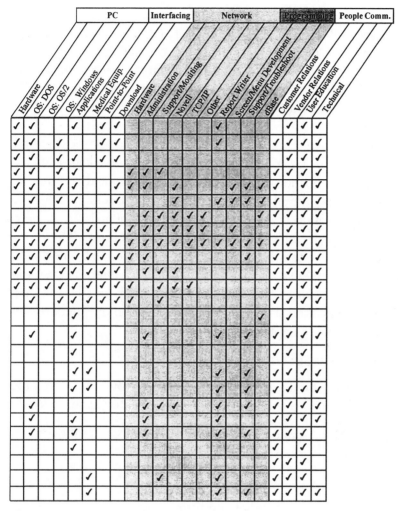

Figure 4.3 *(Continued)*

Standards for technology selection are especially critical because of the need to integrate applications to reduce redundancy between systems and job functions throughout the organization. Integration of data between systems has become a critical success factor for most health care organizations in supporting better data collection and improving the level of patient care. Communication standards such as transmission control protocol/interconnect protocol (TCP/IP) and interface engines now support communication of systems that once operated as islands. It is critical that each organization work with users to define a communication or integration strategy as part of this process and educate users on the importance of adhering to the strategy.

Adherence to an integration strategy also allows an organization to consider basic user communication packages, such as E-mail, which improve the level of organizational communication and productivity of the organization. Users can network personal computers and transfer files if standards are selected for word processing and spreadsheet functions. These may sound like simple solutions, but they are often extremely difficult to implement and maintain because users are accustomed to current packages and may have many years of files on a particular application. For additional information on standards and principles, see Chapter 5: Emerging Standards.

Information Services Budget

The IS budget is a critical component in the overall IS organization analysis. The budget needs to be evaluated at three levels:

- Maintenance of current systems (hardware and applications)

- IS staff salaries

- Planned capital expenditures

The operating budget consists of maintenance and salary expenses. Maintenance of existing systems is usually divided by hardware platform, grouping of applications (financial, clinical, administrative, etc.) and supplies; whereas, the capital budget can be evaluated in terms of the level of investment the organization is prepared to make in new applications and technologies.

The overall IS budget is typically measured as a percentage of total organization revenues. A realistic budget analysis for health care organizations is to weigh the level of spending for IS against the level of automation (application and technology). To evaluate where your organization is in relationship to other health care providers, you can compare your IS budget to that of comparable health care organizations. A comparable health care organization can be selected based on the size and complexity of systems it is maintaining. Specific comparisons are usually made between the percentage of revenues invested in IS and the level of automation and level of resources required to support the organization.

Growth of IS expenditures in the health care industry is expected to accelerate based on the increased demand for information and the technology that is needed to support storage, retrieval, analysis, and communication of shared-patient data. Until recently, hospitals typically spent 2 to 3 percent of their operating budgets on information systems. Manufacturing concerns have been spending 3 to 5 percent, and financial services organizations have been spending 8 to 10 percent. Over the next few years it is expected that health care capital investments will need to increase to implement the new technologies that are available and in demand. Figure 4.4 depicts the typical levels of spending in these industries.

Future expenditures need to be evaluated based on the desired level of automation and the status of current state applications. In many cases the budget analysis will show that an organization has not upgraded existing applications and hardware for several years, requiring an investment in these older technologies to meet changing environmental needs. These weaknesses may require a significant capital investment to correct.

The technology platform(s) that an organization is currently supporting can significantly influence the IS capital budget. In many cases, transaction systems for accounting and billing functions were implemented several years ago and may operate on older platforms that have not been upgraded over time. These platforms may no longer be supported or may not have the ability to be networked or integrated to other applications. In these cases, technology may significantly impact the

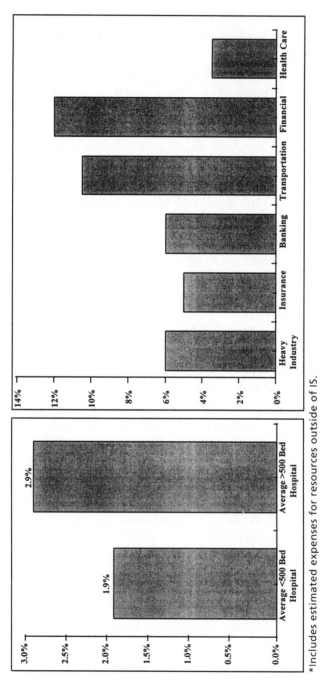

*Includes estimated expenses for resources outside of IS.

Figure 4.4 *Current State: IS Budget as a Percentage of Operating Budget*

capital budget because dollars that could be used to purchase new applications and functionality need to be allocated to hardware upgrades for existing systems. The ideal case is to find a balance between the two in the budget process.

Application Assessment

The application assessment focuses on the current portfolio of applications available throughout the organization. These applications are evaluated based on their ability to support users' current needs and to potentially support future needs or integration with new applications. The application assessment can be divided into two categories:

- Current application portfolio
- Future application needs

The purpose of conducting a current-state application assessment is to analyze the ability of the existing applications to support the core functions, the future-state vision, and the migration to the future-state. The outcome of this process is an understanding of the ability of the existing applications to support current user needs and the future-state vision. Usually this process will result in a list of short-term enhancements that can be made to address functional weaknesses as well as a list of long-term projects that address major functional weaknesses.

Current Application Portfolio

The current application assessment focuses on the portfolio of applications that are supported throughout the organization or enterprise. The assessment should also focus on any applications currently in place that support affiliated lines of business such as long-term care. In the current application assessment, each application is evaluated on the following criteria:

- Ability to support user needs
- Level of satisfaction with the application and vendor

- Age of the application and level of maintenance required to maintain the application

- Technical platform of the application

An understanding of each application and its ability to support users' existing needs is typically gained through the information-gathering process discussed earlier. Also to be considered are the maintenance requirements for the application and technical platforms. Many traditional transaction-based applications were developed over time and do not support integration.

In some cases, organizations have assumed the task of programming maintenance for older applications that are no longer supported by vendors or may have been highly customized to meet specific user needs. The long-term maintenance costs for in-house support of an application may be higher than the cost of replacing the in-house system with a newer system that supports additional functionality. With the quickly changing health care requirements, many organizations with in-house-maintained applications are finding it difficult to keep up with changing regulations.

The result of the current application assessment is an understanding or scorecard of the current application environment as a whole. There is usually a group of applications that support the organization's core business functions (e.g., patient registration, admissions, billing, and general accounting). These core applications need to be evaluated based on their ability to be integrated with other applications and their support of both the current and future business strategies for the organization. An important piece of the planning puzzle is an understanding of the applications users currently have access to in terms of functionality, level of automation, and ability to support reporting needs. Developing a thorough understanding of users' level of sophistication with automation will better support the planning process for a migration plan to the future state. You need to understand where you are coming from in order to map out a path to the future state.

When evaluating existing and future applications, it is important to remember that many enterprises now consist of business units with differing lines of business. The end result is differing application requirements and systems needs that are competing for one set of IS department resources. Also, the traditional health care IS solutions may not apply to all lines of business and affiliations. This is when technology and integration strategies need to be closely evaluated with the application solution.

Future Application Analysis

The future application analysis focuses on applications that will be required to meet the future enterprise needs as defined in the future-state vision. Future application needs are defined based on the business strategies and critical success factors identified through the interview process with senior management and the user departments. Once future systems requirements have been developed, a gap analysis is conducted to determine which applications in the current portfolio will require enhancement or replacement and to what new applications that will need to be implemented.

With the recent changes in the current health care marketplace, several new types of applications have emerged to meet changing health care requirements. These include enterprise systems that support patient registration and access to patient data across multiple entities, computer-based patient records that support collection of patient clinical data for access throughout the health care organization, and managed care systems that support collection of patient data and claims for the capitated health care marketplace. Many vendors are now incorporating these functions into their existing product lines. When evaluating future applications, you should keep in mind the technical platform and level of integration of the current applications. Selecting the best functional application may increase overall maintenance functions if the future systems are not compatible with existing systems. For this reason, the technology and application assessments should be conducted concurrently.

(See Chapter 6: Technology—Architecture and Enablement for a more detailed account of emerging technologies.)

Technology Assessment

To define the migration path to the future state, it is important to focus on the technology that is required to support both current and new applications. Specific areas of focus include:

- Current technology platforms and operating systems

- Integration strategy and connectivity of systems

- Ability to support and migrate to new technologies

Current Technology Assessment

It is becoming increasingly important to establish standards that support and incorporate new technologies as they become proven. This begins with an evaluation of the technology platform for the existing applications and an analysis of its ability to support integration with future applications.

As applications are assessed, the technology platforms and operating systems they operate on must also be assessed. Applications running on old platforms have the potential of requiring more maintenance and can place the organization at risk if the hardware or operating system fails. It is typically very difficult to find people to maintain older technology platforms and operating systems and, therefore, vendors may charge higher fees for maintenance. Also, these systems will most likely not fit into the long-term integration and communication strategy of the organization.

Replacement of older applications can often be a difficult decision because users may be satisfied with the functionality of the applications and processing ability of the system; however, the platform may no longer support the processing needs of the organization. Many times an organization will need to replace a core business system operating on a older platform before implementing new functionality.

Assessment of the Integration Strategy

Integration of information is becoming increasingly important to improve productivity throughout the organization and eliminate redundant functions across departments. This is particularly important with the staff reductions that many organizations have recently been facing.

The integration strategy should address standards for communication protocols for all systems and utilization of interface tools such as an interface engine. The integration strategy must be consistent with the technology standards and is integral to the network strategy selected. The integration strategy must also be flexible enough to support communication with other organizations internal or external to the entity (e.g., third-party payers, physicians' offices, etc.).

A large component of the integration strategy is the analysis of existing networks throughout the organization. With the improvement of network technology, many organizations have local area networks (LANs) implemented within departments to improve the capacity for sharing data within the specific department. This strategy may improve productivity within the specific department but may not support integration with other networks throughout the organization.

It is critical to set networking standards that address the entity or enterprise as a whole to support communication between the entity. A single network protocol will simplify the implementation of standard packages such as E-mail, word processing, and spreadsheet functions that benefit the whole organization.

Future Technology Assessment

As the future state is defined, support for the technology recommended will need to be considered. This relates to the skill mix of the IS staff. It is important to evaluate the skill set required to support the existing and future-state applications and their respective technology platforms as part of the planning process. From this point an education plan is usually developed to support training of existing staff on new technologies, or a hiring plan is executed to recruit additional staff with the specific skill sets in new technologies.

Summary

A realistic assessment of the current IS strengths and weaknesses is critical to a successful migration to the future-state vision. In many cases the current assessment will lead to identification of short term benefits that can be implemented immediately to support enhanced user satisfaction or better operating procedures in the IS department.

The purpose of the current assessment is to gain a thorough understanding of the organizational structure, applications, and technology currently available throughout the organization. In many cases the organization and technology projects may be difficult to define and address with the user community, since they may not see any tangible benefit to the project. However, these projects are just as important as the application projects in developing an IS department that can truly support the current and future needs of the organization.

The next step following the current assessment is to assign implementation priorities to the projects identified in the current state assessment and future-state visioning process and to begin developing a migration strategy to move the organization into the future-state vision.

5

Emerging Standards

Overview

This chapter will focus on how principles and standards guide the organization toward achieving its vision. We will define principles and standards, compare them, then discuss their benefits. While principles are usually specific to an organization, standards are usually objective and market driven. Many of today's standards—open systems, relational database, and so on—affect any CIO in any business but others are unique to the health care industry—Health Level Seven (HL7), American College of Radiology/National Electrical Manufacturers Association (ACR/NEMA), and so on.

Of Principles and Standards

As health care institutions consolidate, they need to merge not only the information technology systems in use by the individual partners but also the principles on which those systems operate. Those principles can be stated as a set of imperatives about the role of information technology within the organization and about the behavior of individuals within the organization with regard to the information technology. Figure 5.1 summarizes the types of principles employed by an organization.

For instance, a general principle in the development of an information system for the entity might be that "business strategy will primarily dictate the selection of a given implementation scenario, not technical considerations."

A user principle might be that "professionals will have access to an intelligent workstation and to the resources (information, computing space, decision support tools, etc.) that they need in order to become more effective."

A principle regarding vendors and development efforts might be that "in-house development will be pursued only when no appropriate off-the-shelf product is available to meet a user's automation requirements."

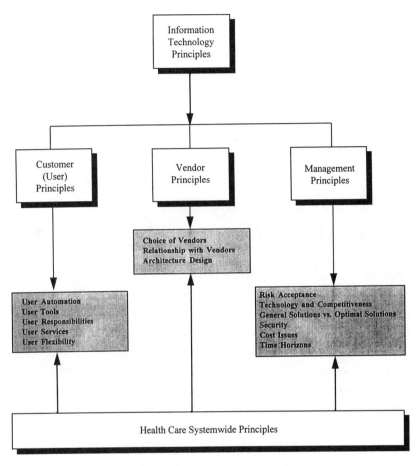

Figure 5.1   *Information Technology Principles*

Another might be that "functionality will drive system selection" (possibly leading to the so-called "best-of-breed" principle).

An entity may, in fact, have dozens of principles.

Only after principles have been agreed on can the organization begin to coalesce around standards. Standards are a set of either/or choices that are often suggested or dictated by the industry or are even de facto by virtue of the marketplace. For instance, the workstation standard for marketing communications firms that produce sophisticated graphics and newsletters is a high-level Macintosh because of its sophisticated graphics capabilities.

A relational data base has become an information technology industry standard. Once an entity has embraced that standard, the particular software used is often dictated by the marketplace—Oracle or Sybase are the most popular. Therefore, we say they have become the de facto standard for the relational data base standard.

The Technologies of Integration

Within a coalescing health care provider network, there will often be multiple overlapping information systems. Tying them together and then allowing the capabilities and capacity for distributed processing is at best a difficult task. Complex networks are required to connect intelligent workstations to multiple serving systems and to connect the serving systems' platforms to each other. In addition, these networks are now extended to geographically distant locations, as seen in Figure 5.2.

Systems

Until the late 1980s health care providers used one of four computer architectures:

■ A mainframe-based computer utilizing the hardware vendor's proprietary operating system—for instance, an IBM mainframe with the MVS (Multiple Virtual Systems) operating system—with programs developed in either Common Business-Oriented Language (COBOL), Assembly Language, or both. Such systems were expensive to buy and maintain, since they needed large facilities and a small army of operators, analysts, and managers.

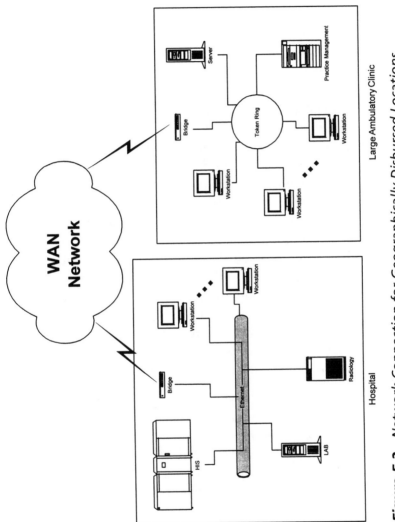

Figure 5.2 *Network Connection for Geographically Disbursed Locations*

91

■ A 32-bit, proprietary super minicomputer, also utilizing a proprietary operating system—for instance, a Digital Equipment Corporation (DEC) VAX series processor with DEC's VMS operating system. Capacity was sacrificed for reduced costs of hardware, facilities, and staff.

■ A super mini utilizing the Massachusetts General Hospital Universal Multi-Programming System (MUMPS), developed in the late 1960s and early 1970s to create a specialized system software environment that included communication, transaction processing, database, and other applications along with the traditional operating software. The downside was the need to purchase or develop in-house application software written in the MUMPS language and using the MUMPS data storage environment.

The use of MUMPS was (and is) not necessarily a bad thing in itself. It does however, present the system's developer with challenges that are otherwise handled by mainstream platform and systems software vendors. For instance, if MUMPS is the operating system, who is providing support for rapidly moving and platform specific technologies such as symmetric multiprocessing and RAID disk storage?

■ An outsource arrangement. Under this architecture the health care organization contracts with a second organization to operate the application. Considerations for this option include reduced risk because of proven implementation and operation strategy and greater control because the health care organization was absolved of all processing responsibilities. However, they became one of many licensees vying for scarce resources for needed customizations, and a premium was paid to have another organization process the transactions.

Perpendicular to the four different architectures, health care provider organizations created information processing services in one of three ways:

- Design and build custom applications utilizing the services of internal programming staff or consultants. A very few institutions were able to turn these systems into products to sell to other institutions, but for the most part they were used solely by the developing organization.

- Have a software or systems solutions vendor build a unique solution for the institution with the intention of turning the solution into a product it could market.

- Purchase a software package designed for another institution along with source code and the right to modify; then customize the package, using in-house or consulting programmers. The purchaser then had a range of additional operations options to choose from. They ranged from running their purchased product in-house with their own employees operating and supporting the systems all the way to using some form of facilities management agreement to run the software at a remote location on resources that were essentially rented from the contracted services provider.

- Purchase a software package and use its built in capabilities to tailor the package as needed. Additional software can be purchased or built to augment the package but the package itself remains "intact" and supported by the package vendor.

The integration of health care provider organizations has created another reason, beyond "best-of-breed," for integration of disparate computer applications and architectures. Hardware, software, and health care industry standards all must be explored when a newly merged institution is deciding which of the various computer systems to discard and which will become the core of its new integrated system.

This is not a trivial task. There are at least three areas that need to be addressed. The first two are effectively the front and back ends of the system. The third is the network that ties the front and back ends together. Taken altogether, these three elements create a distributed computing environment known as client-server architecture, shown in Figure 5.3.

Front End—The User's Application

User solutions are on the front-end. Today this usually means client-server architecture solutions. On the very front end is presentation management and business logic rules. Application users are no longer content with single sessions running on dumb terminals. More and more, users are replacing their terminals with intelligent work stations that provide Graphical User Interfaces (GUIs), the ability for multiple sessions on the same device at the same time, and local processing capabilities. This allows for use of spreadsheet, word processing, database, reporting, and other applications that are clearly superior to

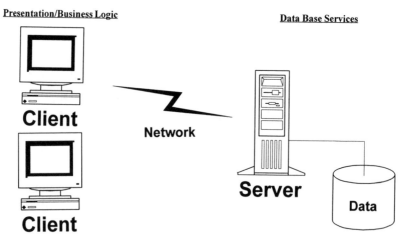

Figure 5.3   Client Server Distributed Computing

similar host- or server-based offerings. The demand for multiple sessions brings particular demands to the workstations themselves, the network, and the host serving platforms.

A complication is that there is not a single standard workstation—or client-server—architecture. The most common workstation is an IBM-compatible PC, but there is also an entrenched core of Macintosh computers, which have software that is incompatible with PCs.

When personal computers were introduced in the early to mid-1980s, users found PC spreadsheet, word processing, E-mail, and other generic office solutions far better than anything they could get from their applications-solutions vendors and computer system suppliers. Since these users already had nonintelligent terminals sitting on their desks, they first needed a way of getting their PCs to act like terminals so they could eliminate the redundant devices. Since the PC could emulate just about any terminal, with the right terminal emulation software, the PC became the retained device.

Desktop computers with graphical user interfaces, which began to proliferate in the late 1980s, added easy-to-understand icons, pop-up and pull-down menus, and drag-and-drop features that were far more understandable than cryptic typed commands. By the first part of the 1990s, the PC had become a major part of most provider institutions' computing operations.

About the same time as the PC and the graphical user interface arrived, the necessary hardware arrived in the form of local area networks (LANs) and central computer systems to create a true distributed computing environment. The workstation could now off-load some of the useful work from the serving host computer system. The serving host system is still best suited for all users of a system. This means the application data bases and possibly the processing logic that is close to this data (e.g., security). The resulting client-server architecture (whether or not it uses what computer experts consider to be "true" client-server applications) provides a wide range of opportunities for implementing distributed computing.

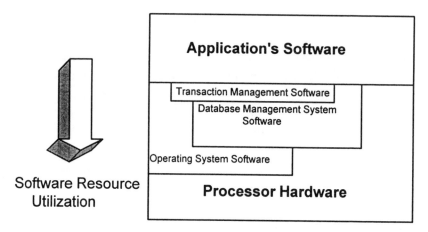

For a system to be truly open, all components under the application's code would have to be interchangeable. In fact, all components must be matched, including the processor hardware. The usual definition of open actually only applies to the API interface between the software components.

Figure 5.4   *Open Systems*

To this day, there is no one standard for client-server architecture, although there is a lot of experience with it, and the architecture has a lot of promise. The first decade of experience also shows that client-server seems to cost far more and take far longer to implement than anyone is ever able to predict at the outset of a development project.

A key decision is whether or not to use what is commonly called open-system architecture. Open systems provide a hardware and system software environment, regardless of supplier, that appears largely the same to applications software, as seen in Figure 5.4. They provide the basis for sets of common tools that can be developed on one system and then relatively inexpensively rehosted onto other systems, providing greater leverage for suppliers and, ultimately, lower costs for customers.

Open systems, however, are not available on all possible combinations of hardware or system software. And they are still proprietary. The trade name UNIX™—the first open system, designed by the Bell Laboratories in the 1970s—is now held by

Novell, and AT&T holds the rights to its System 5.4, which is generally regarded as the feature, function, and application program standard of UNIX. There are hundreds, perhaps thousands, of companies that provide implementations of System 5.4 of UNIX on almost any conceivable computer platform, each with subtle differences. This all must be evaluated before choosing an open-system vendor—indeed, before deciding to use an open system rather than a proprietary system.

Windows, the most popular operating system for the PC—a de facto standard—is not an open system. Only Microsoft Corporation can enhance or maintain Windows. Despite this, Windows, which provides a graphical user interface and the ability to manipulate multimedia, is rapidly becoming the workstation standard in the health care industry.

Back End—The Distributed Data Environment

A number of issues must be considered when integrating the back end database with other information systems. For instance:

- Real-time versus batch (file transfer) interfaces

- Message translation and mapping

- Storage and forwarding of messages

- One-to-many message explosion and many-to-one message implosion

- Message exception handling and correction

- Message recovery

The physical aspects of message-based systems integration are assisted through integration tools such as the so-called interface engine, or translator, in order to facilitate the movement of multiple classes of messages between systems. For instance, you don't just admit patients; you also preadmit, transfer, discharge, update information, cancel admissions, post charges, update the census, and so on. All these messages may come

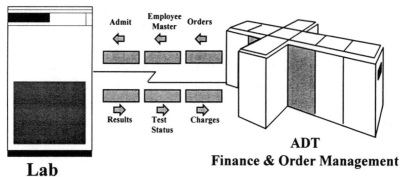

Figure 5.5   *Logical Connections*

from or go to the same physical system. But, as Figure 5.5 shows, these are different messages requiring a logical interface in addition to a physical interface.

Although the interface engine does not eliminate these logical interfaces, it simplifies the typology. All interfaces now become an interface between a sending or receiving system and the interface engine itself. One end of each logical interface is

- Without an interface engine, the number of connections is geometrically proportional to the number of systems

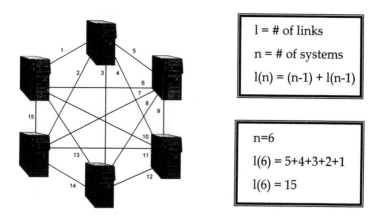

l = # of links

n = # of systems

$l(n) = (n-1) + l(n-1)$

$n=6$

$l(6) = 5+4+3+2+1$

$l(6) = 15$

Figure 5.6   *Physical Connections without an Interface Engine*

now a constant and controllable system. The interface engine is designed to easily adapt to the needs of a source or target system, thus eliminating a stalemate situation where the source and target systems cannot talk to one another, and neither can be changed for technical or economic reasons.

Interface engines also reduce the number of physical connections. Rather than physical connections increasing geometrically with the number of systems connected with an interface engine, the number of connections is n + 1, as shown in Figures 5.6 and 5.7. Finally, interface engines are internal development and operations tools, and include the ability to support:

- A graphical and intuitive development and debugging interface that allows the user to quickly form message structure and correct errors.

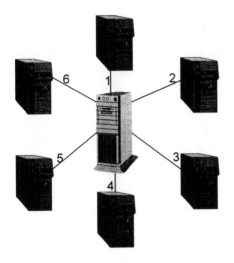

- **The Interface engine changes the geometry**
- **The number of physical connections now equals the number of systems**
- **It can also create other advantages...**

Figure 5.7 *Physical Connections with an Interface Engine*

- Development, test, and live environments on the same or backup platforms.

- A library of communications protocol handlers and previously implemented interfaces that can be used as tool kits.

- Truly scalable and reliable hardware configurations. Interface engines quickly become critical single points of failure within an information systems environment. They need to be at least as reliable and available as the most critical system attached to them.

- The ability to correct and update interface code in a live environment without affecting the operations of other active interfaces.

- Commodity-priced hardware and software components that can be adjusted to fit individual user requirements.

Communications and switching applications, such as interface engines, are particularly inefficient and ineffective on operating systems such as the PC's DOS that effectively slow the processor to the speed of a single communications link. An interface engine's operating system must allow multiple communications links to operate in parallel.

Networks

Networks are the glue that provides the ability to connect systems. Health care information systems are evolving into networks of thousands of devices. The demands on these networks have been significant and this trend will continue. Multimedia, including still and moving images and voice, are being added to the data mix. Diagnostic reference-quality medical images are also starting to appear more often outside of the radiology department. Client-server applications architecture itself can, and usually does, create greater demands on a network. All of these factors are increasing the demands on networks for both bandwidth and utilization.

At the same time, networks themselves are being moved out into the community, state, and country. Users now need, over wide area networks (WANs), the same level of application and device service they previously received inside an institution through local area networks (LANs).

While all of this demand is growing, the U.S. telecommunications industry is also creating new, sophisticated, and complex Wide Area Network technologies, such as Asynchronous Transfer Mode (ATM), to provide local area network-like performance, including such higher-speed technologies as 100-megabits-per-second (mbps) Ethernet networks. At the same time, ATM will be able to carry video conferencing and voice over the same link, using bandwidth only on demand, with reliable guaranteed performance. ATM technology will also find its way to internal networks. Initially, however, it will be a significant new offering from local and long-distance phone companies before the turn of the century.

In the not-too-distant future, cable television lines or direct fiber optic into homes will add to complete the highway. Telephone companies have upgraded the infrastructure between their offices to all fiber in major markets. They will now deploy much higher speed links directly to home or office. Ultimately cable TV operators will also be allowed to compete with phone companies, and both will compete to provide very high bandwidth capabilities to all users, including homes and offices. In any case, the technology and the need both exist. The only doubt is the availability and cost.

Local Area Networks (LANs)

In the early 1980s most information system users gained access to their computer system through a video terminal attached to a dedicated wire that was ultimately attached to a mainframe or super minicomputer system. The information sent to the user was in the form of alphanumeric characters. The typical speed of information transfer was about 1,000 characters per second—the entire screen could be filled within two seconds.

LANs were first considered merely to be a way to make the wiring of computer networks less expensive and more flexible, allowing users to switch terminal connections to different computers without changing any physical wiring simply by using software in the LAN. But fiber optic and other technology has increased LANs' abilities to move information much faster and to transparently share information resources such as disks, printers, and modems.

Today, serving-host computers are able to connect to desktop computers acting as terminals or as client computers. The most obvious need for this occurs when a desktop computer replaces a terminal, and now the user wants an entire file, instead of just a screen, of information deposited onto the local hard disk from the application's host computer system.

The most widely used LAN technologies are categorized by the architecture of the underlying wiring and the way it is used.

Ethernet was originally developed in the 1970s by Xerox's Palo Alto Research Center (PARC). The concept is relatively simple: Basically all LAN devices are attached to a common backbone cable. There are, however, several technical problems with Ethernet in its simplest form. Efforts to make it more robust make it more complicated.

A number of Ethernet standards have been developed by the Institute of Electrical and Electronics Engineers (IEEE) and the International Standards Organization (ISO) with regard to packet formats, addressing, plug compatibility, and cabling. Ethernet standards assume that all users share a common electrical cable and can hence talk or listen over the same cable.

Ethernet operates under a set of rules—Media Access Controls (MAC)—to deal with collisions. In general, if a transceiver (the device that connects to the LAN) detects that it has stepped on another device's signal, they will both back off for a random period of time, then try again. This can slow Ethernet down and is a problem if there is one processor on the Ethernet that has a lot to say, such as sending radiographic images. At the expense of making the network more complicated and expensive, Ethernet can be broken up into addressable segments to get around such problems.

Token Ring is an alternative LAN developed by IBM. It comes in 4- and 16-million-bit per-second versions and conceptually looks like a ring. Token Ring is usually found where an information systems organization got started in LANs while using an IBM mainframe or AS/400 system. Token ring is incompatible with and conceptually very different from Ethernet, but gateways are available to connect a Token Ring LAN to an Ethernet LAN.

Just like Ethernet, Token Ring is not actually wired the way it is conceptually drawn. Token Ring uses hubs to isolate the connection from the ring itself. Token Ring also has a media access method that is deterministic, while Ethernet's is probabilistic. Consequently, it is easier to plan the expected performance of a Token Ring network. No user on a Token Ring LAN can effectively take any more than its fair share of LAN bandwidth. This is accomplished through a somewhat more complex scheme, where every connection node's hub in the network is always active, accepting and passing a token around the ring, and only the processor currently holding the token can use the LAN. All of this, along with smaller market acceptance, makes a Token Ring LAN more expensive than Ethernet.

Wide Area Networks (WANs)

WANs provide the communication capacity that ties information services over a geographically disperse area. Strictly speaking, WANs are required whenever a user's cabling must cross a public right-of-way. Public common carriers are licensed to run cabling over or under public rights of way. In the simple case of a hospital with one building on the other side of the street from its other facilities, a simple right-of-way exception (or waiver) might be granted by a local government or phone company. But institutions with computer systems and users at multiple sites, must use relatively expensive media or equipment (or both) to connect it all together.

Historically, this was done by dial-up services that provided a vehicle for users to log into a host computer from home or office. More complex WANs allowed terminal device users at one location to log into and use remote computer systems with the same performance as users who were local to the host system.

If all information services can be quantified in terms of characters displayed on a screen or printed on a remote printer, then relatively inexpensive services—a few hundred dollars a month—may be all that is required of the WAN. If use of the connectivity is intermittent, then even less expensive dial-up services may be sufficient. But if the on-line integration of LANs is required or if there are large file transfers or multimedia applications, then relatively expensive dedicated high-speed communications services may be required.

Emerging application technologies such as computerized clinical records, document and medical imaging, video conferencing, and voice dictation are all having a significant impact on WAN capacity requirements. In addition, the emergence of client-server environments, whether used by a new vendor-supplied or an in-house-developed application, will place new and very likely severe demands on WAN capacity.

The most typical demand now effectively requires the WAN to extend the LAN between geographic locations. This implies WAN capacities that are 100 to 200 or more times higher than those typically used until the early 1990s. Furthermore, users are beginning to demand, or will demand by the turn of the century, these services in potentially hundreds or even thousands of different geographical locations.

For example, the new computer-based patient record (CPR) system that utilizes client-server technology must be made available to on-call physicians in their homes so they can refer to patient test results and medical history before prescribing treatment over the phone.

Network Operating Systems

Widespread use of networks has created the need for network operating systems. In the simplest sense, a network operating system extends common services, capabilities, and management to all network interconnected users.

Popular products such as Novell's Netware, Banyan's Vines, IBM's LAN Server, Microsoft's LAN Manager, Windows for Workgroups, and Windows/NT Advanced Server are frequently found in institutions with hundreds, or even thousands, of processors and devices. Network operating systems typically run on one or more dedicated server systems that are connected over the same LAN with the user's system. For very small configurations, some peer-to-peer network operating systems are available that effectively allow the network operating system to live in each user's system and eliminate the need for separate network server systems.

Network operating systems primarily rely on the concept of redirection to provide useful and meaningful services to a user. Network servers are used to providing common disk file services, tape services, and printer services transparently to individual workstation users. These facilitate sharing disk files between users and can save money when printers and disk space are carefully managed. Network operating systems also facilitate access to E-mail services, fax services, and shared copies of application software.

Network operating systems have two features that are especially important to information system managers: network management and network security. Network management gives a central authority the ability to monitor activity, capacity, and the overall health of a node or a processing device attached to the network. In order for this to happen, the node must conform to a standard that requires the node to identify itself to the network manager and must respond to certain pre-defined requests for information or action sent by the network management system. The two most popular network management products in use today are IBM's NetView (and NetView/6000 on the IBM RS/6000) and HP's OpenView.

As for network security, reasonably secure environments can be set-up that require users of systems attached to the network, to identify themselves via usernames and passwords before they are allowed access to network resources such as disk directories and printers. In addition, the specific resources can be limited by username. Thus even though the PC itself may not be a secured device, the access of any given user to the network through an unsecured PC can be limited and monitored through centrally managed network security.

Databases

Databases are also part of integration and are distributed within many new client-server applications. It is not unusual to see a vendor offer both a central database for information that must be truly centralized as well as local workstation databases. These decisions are usually made to enhance performance and flexibility to the user sitting at the workstation.

In order to get predictable reliable performance and data integrity, it is essential that an information services department understand the data that needs to be managed and how it might be managed by applications systems. An institutional data model that is a dynamic part of the organization's information planning and operations is a requirement. Without a current data model, it is impossible to understand the real effectiveness of new systems that are being planned. It is also impossible to understand the effect that a new application will have on the operation of the existing system.

Emerging clinical data repository products should be particularly studied. These products are designed to store and display or report just about any information that might exist within a health care organization. Most systems are actually based on one or more relational databases and have a particularly complex structure that is needed to access, in an efficient manner, all of this information. In order to develop and implement these systems, the vendors have developed their own data models as a basis for building the relational structures that actually hold the information in the relational database management system.

These data models are built on a series of compromises to provide:

- User extendibility

- Quick performance for on-line use

- Efficient data storage to accommodate data structures that can have multiple occurrences

- Normalization to optimize the writing and updating processes

- De-normalization to minimize access time

There is no one correct model. Any vendor's model may or may not fit well with a health care organization's defined—or implied—data model. A health care organization should not embark on decisions about interfaces, processes, or content without a clear understanding of the similarities or differences between these data models.

Database Architecture

Any health care enterprise processes and stores an extremely large amount of diverse and complex data. In an ideal situation, all of this data could be kept in one place and accessed in a common way by all applications. This idealized environment would have only one database system that owns all data. When any piece of data needed to be updated or deleted, there would be only one location that would have to be changed. This full normalization of data would also ensure that space is not wasted by keeping redundant copies of the same data in multiple locations.

But the real world cannot tolerate this homogeneity. Health care enterprises are diverse organizations. The larger the enterprise, the less likely that the information services department has the time, focus, or political clout to create or specify and provide the applications solutions that all users must use. There is also a variety of user departments in a health care organization with various needs for computer automation support, and these departments often seek, sometimes on their own, a best-of-breed solution from different software vendors.

Each software solution acts as an independent island of data and expects to manage its data as if the data existed nowhere else in the provider organization. For example, a member's registration system, orders communications system, and billing system, all need to know basic demographic information about a patient (name, date of birth, address, etc.). As originally developed and independently installed, all systems collect the data independently, which leads to redundancies and inconsistencies.

In order to solve this problem, an explicit effort is needed to integrate the information between disparate systems. Electronic messages need to be developed and exchanged between these systems whenever an event occurs that adds or modifies data that exists in multiple places. Going one step further, messages can be used to request information from other systems rather than storing a redundant copy of a seldom-used piece of information on a local system.

Broken out individually, this concept requires hundreds of separate message interfaces. Fortunately, the physical interconnections between the processing systems can all be handled within the LAN. Several different types of message exchanges can take place between the individual host processing systems using the same LAN connections. The messages themselves are, however, quite complex. The exact information required can vary greatly, depending on the capabilities of an individual vendor's applications.

Interface Standards

Any health care enterprise struggles with the problems of data integration. Conceptually, we would like to get the functional benefits of best-of-breed solutions while maintaining the simple data architecture of a single data base. Although there is no simple solution to this dichotomy, there are methods and tools that can address it.

In the simplest analysis, application messaging standards are some of the tools that help separate systems work together. This is an extremely broad statement that could refer to literally thousands of different standards within a single implementation. Most of the applicable standards involve issues that, typically, do not have to be dealt with by anyone except the engineer who designs a specific system.

Data issues are not so easily standardized. The data needs of an individual health care institution or enterprise are based on the business and clinical process in use. The business of providing health care implies procedures that caregivers, administrators, and others follow in order to provide care to a patient. There are no standardized business processes for health care. With the possible exception of a single corporate entity that operates virtually identical delivery, there is no standardization of detailed business or clinical processes. Therefore, for now, there is no standardization for data architecture and methods for the information systems that support these business and clinical processes.

Messaging Standards

Messaging standards can exist as a way of describing and supporting a large part of an organization's de facto data model that is derived from empirical use of data. Data processing standards that cover topics such as operating systems, database systems, query languages, communications protocols, and so on, certainly provide a framework for data integration. Application messaging standards—communications standards that reside at the seventh layer of the International Standards Organization's open systems interconnect model—provide assistance in standardizing the way applications communicate information to each other. At the very least, messaging standards can provide a bridge to facilitate communication between systems.

Messaging standards imply that the communicating systems work from data that is of identical process, structure, and form. This means that the messages are used between systems for predefined and expected reasons; the messages themselves are understandable to both systems, even though the actual data may be encoded (e.g., SNOMED). It must be understood, however, that there are still several shortcomings that prevent the sought after plug-and-play environment. These include:

- Different institutions have different process events that cause data to move between systems. For instance, one institution's admission may be another institution's combined-member registration-and-encounter transaction.

- Communications environments require that multiple hardware and software properties match identically. The fact that both systems are attached to an Ethernet, for example, is not enough to affect communications between two applications programs running on two different systems.

- Communications and switching applications are particularly inefficient and ineffective on operating systems, such as the PC's disk operating system, that effectively slow the processor to the speed of a communications link and do not allow multiple communications links to operate in parallel.

- Data representation must be common between systems. For example, patient name on one system might be a string of 60 characters, but in another system it might be a component data type consisting of 6 strings, each with a maximum length of 48 characters ordered in a particular way.

- An agreement on the messaging standard required data items, as opposed to optional data items, must exist between systems.

Organizations That Set Standards

A number of health care standards organizations exist today to define the needed message standards for particular domains. In general, these organizations are neither redundant nor overlapping. Most are members of the American National Standards Institute (ANSI) or are currently moving to become members of ANSI. All are members of and working with ANSI's Health Information Standards Planning Panel (HISPP) to establish an ANSI Health Care Standards Board.

American National Standards Institute (ANSI)

Health care messaging standards are far behind those of many other industries. It is much easier to define a message to communicate a travel itinerary, purchase order, or funds transfer than to communicate a standard message for prescribing the administration of a pharmaceutical for a patient in an acute-care facility.

There are, however, a number of organizations developing message standards.

The American National Standards Institute (ANSI), a for-profit membership organization founded in 1918, coordinates over 11,000 voluntary standards for a variety of industries. ANSI also represents the United States in international standards groups such as the United Nations International Standards Organization (ISO).

In health care, ANSI has created the Health Information Systems Planning Panel (HISPP) to serve as an umbrella organization to coordinate activities of all who participate in or are interested in development of health care-related computer messaging standards.

American College of Radiology/National Electrical Manufacturers Association (ACR/NEMA)

The American College of Radiology (ACR) and the National Electrical Manufacturers Association (NEMA), are professional and trade organizations, respectively, that have developed the health care standards for imaging communication.

The ACR/NEMA standards define messages for the exchange of image data as well as the originating equipment specifications, patient study and visit data needed to provide the context for images.

The organization's digital image communications (DICOM) standard has international acceptance and is widely used for communication within a radiology department between digital modality equipment and picture archival and communications systems (PACS). The current version uses an object-model-based approach and defines an application of the Open Systems Interconnect (OSI) protocol stack, a TCP/IP protocol stack and an older proprietary ACR/NEMA protocol stack.

ASC X12N

X12 is an ANSI Accredited Standards Committee, which defines electronic data interchange (EDI) standards in the United States across all industries. Insurance industry standards (the umbrella for health care standards) are within X12N, which deals with several transaction sets that relate to computer-to-computer communications that might take place between a health care provider institution and payer organization. ASC X12 produces the standards themselves, and implementation guidelines are written by the Health Industry Business Communications Council (HIBCC), the Work Group on Electronic Data Interchange (WEDI), and others.

American Society of Testing Materials (ASTM)

ASTM has produced a number of health care-related messaging standards.

ASTM is composed of over 141 committees and health care is organized under the E31 and E32 committee and subcommittees. These groups have, and continue to define standards for results reporting, observations, vocabularies, rules syntax, waveform images, computerized patient records, community health information networks, etc.

HL7

HL7 is an ANSI-Accredited Standards Organization that produces messaging standards related to activities that traditionally occur within a health care delivery organization. Version 2.2 of HL7, published in December 1994, defines messages that deal with a number of areas, including:

- Patient demographics and insurance information for such areas as admissions, discharges, transfers, scheduling, and registration.

- Clinical orders and results reporting (coordinated with ASTM) which includes lab, pharmacy, blood bank, radiology, and dietary orders.

- Financial charges associated with an item or service.

- Master file updates to provide a vehicle for keeping distributed master files synchronized.

- A message to communicate a generalized query from one system to another.

Version 2.3 is expected to be published in mid-1996 and to include messages to support scheduling, episode-of-care management, managed care membership information, chart tracking and completion, immunization, and physician referrals.

Institute of Electrical and Electronic Engineers (IEEE)

IEEE is one of the world's largest professional organizations. The Medical Data Interchange Committee (MEDIX) has, as its focus, the building of health care messaging standards based on computability with ISO's OSI model. The Medical Information Buss (MIB) provides a standard for communications between bedside instruments and health care information systems.

IEEE is also the health care secretariat for data modeling standards in health care. IEEE has coordinated an effort with participation from all of the other groups to create industry specific common data meta models and data model examples.

National Council for Prescription Drug Programs (NCPDP)

In existence since 1978, NCPDP provides a standard for use between retail pharmacies, pharmacy benefits management companies, pharmaceutical wholesalers, and manufacturers, including standards for retrieving benefits information and communicating drug stock use and formulary information.

Standards Influencers

In addition to organizations that develop standards, a number of other organizations, including many arms of the federal government, set policy or take positions that affect the development of standards. These organizations include the Department of Health and Human Service's Health Care Financing Administration (HCFA), the Food and Drug Administration (FDA), the Agency for Health Care Policy and Research (AHCPR), and the General Accounting Office (GAO).

The Work Group on Electronic Data Interchange (WEDI), chartered in 1990 by then Secretary of Health and Human Services, Dr. Louis Sullivan, has produced reports to Congress encouraging use of health care information standards, specifically, ASC X12's EDI standards. WEDI is now reorganizing itself into a private standards advocacy group.

The Computer-based Patient Record Institute (CPRI) was created by an initiative growing out of a National Academy of Sciences commissioned study that was performed by the Institute of Medicine (IOM). This study clearly indicated that there is no clear definition of a CPR, the codes and vocabularies included in medical records, security and confidentiality issues and answers, or any sort of general industry or public agreement on these issues. CPRI has been formed to address these issues.

Much of their work will give direction to the health care standards organizations.

Summary

The CIO in a health care enterprise must be cognizant of a number of standards, both those set by organizations seeking to make uniform health care information messaging and those de facto standards that exist more generally in the world of hardware and software for any business operating today.

But before the CIO can even worry about standards, he or she must be clear about the principles the health care organization develops regarding information technology and its use.

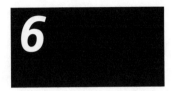

6

Technology— Architecture and Enablement

Overview

A number of new technologies are emerging in the marketplace that hold significant promise for reducing costs and increasing quality. These technologies do not focus on supporting departmental needs but aim to serve the needs of the entire organization. Their purpose is not strictly to automate existing processes but to enable new processes or support new functionality.

Like any technology, however, they are not solutions in and of themselves. These new technologies require clear objectives, management support, and process innovation in order to demonstrate value. Without these factors, they are simply high-cost technologies.

Computer-Based Patient Record Systems[1]

Over the last decade there has been a slow progression in the health care industry toward the computer-based patient record (CPR). Over the last few years a number of vendors have begun offering products that represent real progress toward functional computer-based patient record systems. These products are being designed to interact with caregivers, giving them the ability to place orders, retrieve patient information, and monitor patient care in a way that is more efficient and effective than in a manual, paper-based environment. These products generally require an extensive infrastructure of ancillary systems to support data capture and a network of end-user workstations for convenient access.

Value of a Computer-Based Patient Record System

The computer-based patient record system serves two funda-mental purposes. First, the CPR system is a tool for clinicians, automating much of the paper-intensive processes surrounding care delivery. Specifically, a CPR system can:

- Make access to patient information easy enough so that care providers will choose to use the CPR system over the paper record.

- Enable physicians to directly enter orders into the system.

- Provide the ability to place orders based on predefined clinical pathways.

- Perform conflict checking, duplicate checking, and identify alternative, more cost-effective therapies— providing immediate feedback to the system user.

- Expedite access to results information.

- Provide quick and easy access to longitudinal patient information.

- Provide a common user interface for accessing patient information.

- Convey patient information in a comprehensive, inte-grated manner rather than by departmental orientation.

- Alert designated care givers, based on test results, by pager, fax, printer, or electronic mail.

Second, the CPR system can be used by health care admin-istrators to help manage the care-delivery process. Depending on the types of information collected, a CPR system can provide the ability to assess clinical outcomes and support development of clinical pathways—activities that are becoming increasingly important in light of a reformed health care industry.

Profile of a Computer-Based Patient Record System

A functioning CPR system consists of three main components: the database, the gateway, and the front end. These components are illustrated in Figure 6.1 and explained in detail below.

Gateway

The gateway sends and receives data from external applications and formats the data to match the data model or protocol of the receiving component. The gateway may reside on the same hardware platform as the database or it may reside on a stand-alone computer. Depending on the type of messages being received from the applications, the gateway may be a very simple loading program or it may be a sophisticated application-level gateway or interface engine with the ability to reformat and route delimiter-based messages between applications.

A simple gateway would send and receive already-formatted, fixed-length messages from applications along custom-developed, point-to-point interface links. In this case the data stream, generally, is already formatted to match the

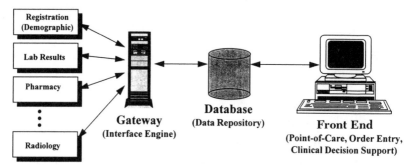

Figure 6.1   *Computer-Based Patient Record System*

database configuration, and the gateway simply loads the data directly into the clinical database.

A more sophisticated gateway/interface engine receives both fixed and variable-length messages, reformats and retransmits the messages to other applications, and sends a formatted copy of the message to the database for storage. In some cases the gateway/interface engine component is offered by the CPR system vendor as an integral part of the CPR system. In other cases the interface engine component is purchased from a separate interface engine vendor.

Based on short- and long-term information systems plans for an institution, the ability to easily configure and modify the gateway may be an important consideration. A user-friendly and easy-to-change gateway/interface engine is very important for organizations involved in consolidation activities.

Database

The database component stores the patient data and, in some cases, manages field-level security for accessing information. The database component consists of a relational database management system (RDBMS) based on either a stand-alone hardware platform or on a platform that is shared with the gateway/interface engine or other applications. For CPR systems, relational databases are preferred over hierarchical and network databases due to the flexibility and relative standardization available in RDBMSs. Relational databases are much easier to tune because indexes and tables can be modified without requiring changes to the related application programs. This makes relational databases ideally suited for client-server environments where performance is sometimes difficult to predict and tuning may be required to optimize performance or to change the underlying data model. Additionally, the ease of data access via structured query language (SQL) and the availability of third-party software packages such as executive information systems make relational databases the flexible type of technology that many organizations require.

Two major issues within the database component must be considered when buying or building a CPR system. First, the RDBMS (Oracle, Ingres, Sybase, DB2, etc.) that manages the data dictates the ability to scale and expand the database in the future, both in overall storage size and in number of tables. The RDBMS also has an impact on performance; and depending on how the CPR system is used, performance can be the most difficult issue to deal with during implementation.

The second issue is the data model. The data model defines the types of information stored and relationships between different sets of information. The data model will have the largest impact on performance and future expandability. Issues include normalization of data and use of indexes. Normalization refers to the way data is arranged in tables in the database and indexes are used to access data based on different search fields. For example, indexing a table to provide the ability to look up a patient by last name, patient ID, phone number, attending physician, referring physician or ward would require additional indexes, which could adversely affect performance. On the other hand, performing queries on fields that are not indexed is CPU intensive and can severely degrade performance. Tuning may be required and limitations should be defined in order to ensure satisfactory response times.

Front End

The front-end component of the CPR system provides the ability to retrieve data from the database and enter orders into the system using a format that is meaningful, efficient, and easy to use. The front end consists of software that resides on a workstation and interacts with the database in a client-server relationship. Depending on requirements, the front end may be written in various third-generation computer languages (3GL) such as COBOL, C, C++, or SmallTalk; or it may be written in a fourth-generation language (4GL) such as Lotus Notes, Powerbuilder, Enfin, Forte, or Dynasty. It may be developed using a computer-aided software engineering (CASE) tool such as ADW, IEF, or Oracle CASE.

The way the front end is engineered has two main effects. The first area affected is system performance. While it is much easier and faster to develop applications using fourth-generation languages or CASE tools, you'll find they can contribute a level of overhead that may slow system response. Conversely, writing applications entirely in a 3GL consumes time and resources and can be more difficult to maintain. An alternative approach sometimes involves developing prototypes in a CASE or 4GL environment to gain physician acceptance, then rewriting the back-end in a 3GL to enhance performance.

The second area affected by front-end engineering may be the most important aspect of the CPR system—system usability. A system that enables staff to shuffle orders or results around more quickly, although valuable, is limited in its ability to change the manner in which business is conducted. But a system that directly interacts with clinicians holds more value than one that is obtained by merely speeding up the current process. Providing clinicians with direct access to sophisticated CPR functionality can result in lower error rates, more complete documentation reduced duplicate orders, and overall higher quality of care.

This is why the front end that is developed must be easy to use and friendly to busy clinicians who have many responsibilities and may not have much time for training sessions. Data access must be simple and intuitive. The front end must also allow some level of customization in order to adapt to different specialties and work styles. The front end should also offer power users the ability to use the system quickly and efficiently.

While the front end does not have to be developed in a graphical environment, use of a graphical environment greatly increases the chances of success. In a study commissioned by Microsoft and Zenith Data Systems,[2] productivity was measured for experienced and inexperienced users in both graphical user interface and nongraphical environments. They found that the GUI users:

- Completed 35 percent more tasks than non-GUI users in the same time.

- Correctly completed 91 percent of their tasks (non-GUI completed 74 percent).

- Correctly completed 58 percent more tasks per unit time.

- Experienced less frustration and fatigue.

- Felt more comfortable exploring the machine and learning new tasks.

This higher level of success, however, is not without cost. A GUI environment requires more processing power and more programming support due to the added complexity of the system. Further, many IS shops do not yet have the resources needed to fully support GUI technology.

State of the Market

CPR systems will have to evolve through several generations before they truly support the vision of a paperless environment. First-generation computer-based patient record systems focus on results reporting only. Information from ancillary systems is collected in the database, providing easy access to the information in a meaningful and comprehensive manner. While these systems can be useful, they do not significantly alter existing processes, and therefore do not offer the opportunity for extensive process reengineering that more robust second-generation products can offer.

Most vendor products on the market today are in this second-generation development stage. A listing of some vendors who are offering CPR products is in Figure 6.2. Many of these

Ameritech (AKD) - CareWindows   Cerner - OCF & Powerchart
Emtek   Epic - Epicare
HBOC   HealthVision - CareVISION
IDX   MedicaLogic - Logician
Oacis Healthcare Systems   Oceania - Wave
Sirius - MedMaster   SMS - LCR, Care Center
Sunquest - SCPR   Systematics (TDS)
Win2

Figure 6.2   *Examples of CPR Vendors*

vendors have designed their products around the acute-care setting and are expanding to the ambulatory setting. Other vendors that specialize in ambulatory or group practice information systems have built their CPR systems around the ambulatory care setting, supporting different needs and a slightly different market.

Second-generation products will provide order-entry capabilities with clinical decision-support functionality and automated critical pathways. Physicians will be able to authorize or modify predefined orders based on the critical pathway. Clinicians will also be able to enter patient information directly into the system. Clinical decision-support functionality will automatically review the order and identify possible conflicts, duplicates, or alternative therapies. Several vendors listed in Figure 6.2 are working on this type of second-generation functionality.

Computer-based patient record systems are one of the most important developments in health care information technology today. CPR systems are multidepartment, multidisciplinary, and multifacility, which opens the window for significant gains in efficiency, quality, and productivity. And although these systems may not immediately support a 100 percent paperless environment, they support more important strategic goals of lower cost, improved quality, and better access.

Health Information Networks

A health information network (HIN) provides the means for electronically sharing information needed to support the health care financing and delivery process. An HIN can offer a number of benefits to participating organizations, including reduced administrative overhead and better access to clinical and financial information. However, as with many new strategies and technologies, a number of obstacles are impeding current efforts to implement HINs.

Value of a Health Information Network

Healthcare organizations today are searching for ways to gain competitive advantage. Three fundamental strategies for doing this are increasing the quality and efficacy of health care delivery, reducing the number of unnecessary procedures and tests, and reducing administrative overhead. As explained below, a health information network can benefit an organization by supporting each of these three strategies.

- *Increase the quality and efficacy of health care delivery.* A health information network can make a broad range of current and historical information available to caregivers when and where they need it. Using the network, caregivers have access to test results from other partner organizations. Furthermore, caregivers have the ability to retrieve this information in their own offices or other predefined locations. Timely access to a broad range of information enables care teams to provide more effective care to their patients.

- *Reduce the number of unnecessary procedures and test for quicker initiation of therapy.* By providing access to a broad range of information, a health information network can support efforts to reduce the number of unnecessary tests. By reviewing a patient's profile, caregivers can easily determine if an order is duplicative. If the network includes decision-support functionality, caregivers could be notified of possible complications or more efficient courses of treatment.

Additionally, a health information network can help reduce the number of unnecessary procedures by providing physicians access to on-line medical libraries and current medical guidelines. Caregivers who have access to the information they need are better able to make informed decisions and provide more effective and efficient care.

■ *Reduce administrative overhead.* A primary mission of a health information network is to reduce administrative overhead and human error associated with moving information between organizations and individuals. Currently a significant amount of repetitive information is moved between organizations. Costs are incurred as staff at each organization individually handle documents and other items as they are routed to their final destinations. Fully standardizing information and moving it electronically significantly reduces the need for frequent human intervention and reduces the costs associated with errors and nonvalue-added activities.

To quantify the savings related to moving standard data sets electronically, the Workgroup on Electronic Data Interchange (WEDI) formed the Technical Advisory Group within its Financial Implications Subcommittee.[3] An April 1993 white paper by the group summarized estimated savings that would be realized if common transactions were fully standardized and exchanged electronically. Figure 6.3 is a summary of the group's estimates.

These figures represent the estimated benefits only from reducing administrative burden faced by most health care

Transaction	*Annual Gross Savings (Millions)*		
	Low End		High End
Enrollment	$ 192	-	$ 393
Eligibility	156	-	338
Referral/Authorization	167	-	176
Appointing/Scheduling	47	-	47
Prescription Ordering	679	-	679
Test Order/Results	294	-	294
Materials Management	2,558	-	4,036
Medical Records	5,100	-	5,100
Claims Submission	5,217	-	9,297
Coordination of Benefits	418	-	598
Claims Inquiry	111	-	111
Payment & Remittance	1,065	-	1,164
TOTAL	$16,004	-	$22,233

Figure 6.3   *WEDI Estimates for Administrative Savings*

organizations. While the figures are significant, they still do not encompass elements that are typically more difficult to measure, such as the cost savings related to higher quality care and a healthier population. It is these less tangible elements that will ultimately prove to be the major benefits of an HIN.

Obstacles Impeding Health Information Networks

As information technology and industry standards continue to mature, health information networks will become more feasible and practical. However, a number of nontechnical obstacles still exist that impede the adaptation of networks as a primary means for moving health-related information between organizations. A few of the more significant obstacles are:

■ *Cost.* The cost of linking health care organizations into a health network is one of the most significant obstacles impeding HINs. Developing electronic links may require capital investment to update legacy systems that were not designed to generate the standards-based messages required for community linkages, depending on the ownership model. Other costs may include standard transaction fees as well as the costs of telecommunications hardware and services.

■ *Competition.* Competition is an issue for health information networks serving communities or collaborative initiatives. Health care organizations may be apprehensive about investing in a project. Issues raised typically include network ownership and governance and sharing of potentially strategic information. In the health care industry, several different approaches for structuring HINs are emerging that support different ownership and information-sharing objectives. The optimal approach for a health information network depends on the individual characteristics of the project.

■ *Security and privacy.* In an HIN, security and privacy issues are addressed by implementing thorough security procedures and permitting access to information only to those who need the information. Patients must provide authorization in order for their records to be accessed through the network. Additionally, patient information can be authorized only for specific caregivers and, if desired, for specific windows of time and specific locations. Standard methods for addressing security and privacy issues are currently being defined by several national organizations.

However, even with stringent security and control mechanisms in place, there is still worry. Frequent stories about computer hackers breaking into extremely secure systems and the potential for accessing large volumes of information makes security a high-profile issue.

■ *Standards.* Although lack of clear standards is an obstacle, many current efforts are breaking this down. In some areas, standardization efforts are new and more effort is required to reach consensus within the industry. In other areas, such as claims processing, standards are well developed and savings are already being realized by organizations employing them. Although significant work is still required, progress continues to be made. The rate of progress in establishing standards will very likely increase in the next few years as the need to efficiently share information increases.

■ *Legislation and regulation.* Legal issues remain as obstacles to HINs. This barrier can be more difficult to address due to the length of time required to make changes to the environment. Thus far, however, legal issues have not proven to be major obstacles to HINs. Research is required to identify specific legal obstacles that may be encountered in individual communities.

In order to make a health information network successful, all major obstacles must be addressed. Many in the health care industry are optimistic that the obstacles facing HINs can be eliminated or at least minimized. In many cases, perceived obstacles will be minimized or eliminated through a straightforward educational process.

Other obstacles can be minimized by building a health information network using an evolutionary approach. Functionality may be added incrementally to allow participating organizations time to enhance existing systems needed to incorporate new capabilities.

Profile of a Health Information Network

A health information network is an innovative combination of services, products, and technology that enables organizations

Clinical	Financial	Administrative
Medical Records (Transfer)	Claim Processing Transaction	Patient Eligibility Information
Orders	- Claim Submission	Patient Preregistration
- Lab	- Claim Status	Benefits Information
- Prescription	- Claim Remittance Advice	Precertification Requirements
- Radiology	- Coordination of Benefits	Referral Processing
- Consultation	- Claim Adjudication	Insurance Plan Enrollment
Results	Financial Settlement	Patient Appointment Scheduling
- Lab	- Electronic Funds Transfer	Supply Orders
- Radiology	- Credit Card Transactions	Utilization Review
- Pharmacy		
Transcription Management		
Medical Libraries		
Knowledge Databases		
Patient Census		
Teleradiology/Telemedicine		

Figure 6.4   *Information Transmitted by a HIN*

to exchange clinical, financial, and administrative information electronically with other designated organizations. Much of the information is currently transferred between organizations via paper document, telephone, or fax; and information that is currently transferred electronically is via redundant, nonstandard networks and computer equipment. Figure 6.4 lists the types of information that can be transmitted electronically on a health information network.

The range of information that can be carried by a network is large, and, accordingly, many organizations within the regional area may be involved. Figure 6.5 illustrates many of the different types of organizations that may be involved in a health information network.

Emerging Strategies

Many vendors are entering the marketplace to support HIN strategies. The vendors offer a diverse set of approaches for meeting needs. The diversity in approaches stems from the diversity in vendor backgrounds. Below is a summary of a few of the various approaches. A partial listing of vendors offering HIN solutions is listed in Figure 6.6.

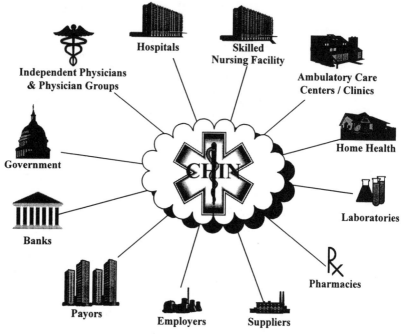

Figure 6.5 *Participants in a HIN*

Network Driven

Most of the HIN solutions on the market are network-driven solutions. Many vendors that offer solutions have origins in telecommunications or electronic data interchange (EDI). Telecommunications companies, in general, are always searching for ways to increase traffic over their networks. (This also is why they subsidize telemedicine pilots so heavily.) EDI

ActaMed Corp.	Ameritech
CyData	Electronic Data System
Equifax	GE Information Systems
GTE Health Systems Inc.	Health Communication Services (HCS)
Health Data Exchange (HDX)	Integrated Medical Systems (IMS)
Integrated System Solutions Corp. (ISSC)	Med Power Inc.
NEIC and value added networks (VANs)	

Figure 6.6 *Examples of HIN Vendors*

vendors, generally, are searching for ways to increase their market share and already have the infrastructure in place to support expanded EDI transaction sets. Other solutions are spin-offs of proprietary networks originally built to serve payer or provider organizations. The products and services have been spun off into independent companies in order to market the solution to other organizations.

These network-driven solutions focus on the network providing the means for moving information between payers and providers. Some solutions focus on providing the connectivity between existing applications. For example, a practice management system may generate billing information that is transmitted over the network to a claims clearinghouse or directly to a payer. In this case the network vendor is only offering the network connectivity as a service. The network vendor does not supply either the practice management system software or the payer software.

For clinical information, however, this is not an option because most practice management applications cannot receive and process clinical information from an outside source. (Most cannot process clinical information at all.) Therefore, for transmission of clinical information and some financial information, the solution is for the vendor to build the front-end workstation software that will reside in the physician's office. The front-end software is essential for the solution to work and is an inherent part of the service offering.

Practice Management System Driven

Several vendors of practice management systems (PMS) are integrating networking capabilities into their practice management systems. This represents a logical progression of electronic claims capabilities that many practice management vendors are beginning to offer. The advantage of this approach is that it offers an integrated solution to physician practices that are already using PMS software. Initial focus is the link with payers to provide claims, eligibility, and referral processing. Second-generation EDI capabilities will focus on connectivity to hospitals and other facilities for clinical information.

Information Superhighway

An alternative approach to moving information between organizations is via the information superhighway. Information services such as America Online and CompuServe offer the infrastructure necessary to move information between offices or facilities. The advantages these services offer are ease of implementation, security features built into the system, and a billing system that tracks individual usage. The Internet may also prove to be a viable option in the future.

Some examples today dispatch transactions over the Internet as E-mail messages. These packages take advantage of the Internet's peer-to-peer connectivity to provide users with the advantages of EDI without incurring the third-party overhead of value-added networks. The most significant issue in this approach is security. One solution is to license RSA Data Security's public key encryption standard to secure the data packets as they are transported over the unsecured Internet.

Information Technology for Managed Care

Defining the scope of information technology for managed care is a significant task. The challenge stems from the confusion surrounding managed care itself. Managed care means many things to many people, and even industry experts concede that managed care cannot be defined concisely. Peter Kongstvedt, in *The Managed Health Care Handbook,* highlights the confusion of the term in his definition for managed care:

A regrettably nebulous term. At the very least, is a system of health care delivery that tries to manage the cost of health care, the quality of that health care, and access to that care. Common denominators include a panel of contracted providers that is less than the entire universe of available providers, some type of limitations on benefits to subscribers who use non-contracted providers, and some type of authorization system. Managed health care is actually a spectrum of systems, ranging from so-called managed indemnity, through PPOs, POS, open panel HMOs, and closed panel HMOs. For a better definition, the reader is urged to read this book [*The Managed Health Care Handbook*] and formulate his or her own.

This confusion, however, has not stopped the health care information systems industry from pressing forward. Many health care technology professionals are already familiar with contract management systems or claims payment or capitation systems constructed around managed care tenets. Individual perceptions of managed care come from the variety of perspectives within the delivery system. The perspective may be from the provider side, payer side, employer side, or member side. Figure 6.7 illustrates the different perspectives from which managed care may be viewed.

Each perspective of managed care encompasses its own set of technologies that are generally referred to as managed care systems. This is because each individual in the care continuum perceives managed care technology as the new system that has arrived because of managed care. Therefore, many caregivers perceive clinical pathway systems as managed care systems. Hospital administrators consider contract management systems managed care systems, and payers view claims and encounter processing systems as managed care systems. Although all of these types of systems may be called managed care systems, they clearly support different needs and different types of organizations.

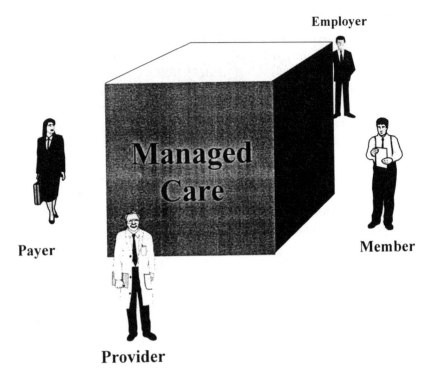

Figure 6.7 *Managed Care Perspective*

Consequently, the term managed care information system is ambiguous and cannot be used to describe any one category of information technology. The real task then is to identify the different types of technology that directly support managed care tenets. These technologies generally support niche needs within a managed care organization or integrated delivery system. Combined with existing legacy systems they support the entire managed care process.

Scope of Managed Care

For managed care systems that receive a fixed per-member per-month (PMPM) premium there is a clear incentive to identify any opportunity that may provide a strategic edge. Managed care organizations, therefore, must address the full spectrum of operations and care delivery to be competitive. This spectrum includes

Health plan services

Members/consumers

Employers

Primary-care physicians

Specialists

Inpatient care

Outpatient care

Ancillary services

Therapeutic services

Emergency department

Skilled nursing facilities

Dental care

Vision

Home care

Behavioral health

Substance abuse

Durable medical equipment

This full continuum is illustrated in Figure 6.8. Along this continuum there is a range of services and products that are needed to help control quality and costs, and facilitate access. Some technologies are required in order to support basic core requirements of a health plan. Other technologies, such as technologies for demand management, support more strategic initiatives. The following sections describe the range of functions

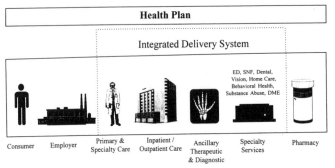

Figure 6.8   *The Continuum of Care*

being addressed by managed care organizations and some of the technologies that support those functions.

Core Health Plan Services

For health plans or payers the core managed care system is a system that supports claims and encounter processing according to contractual arrangements. These systems are also designed to support referral and precertification processing, capitation, risk pools, and enrollment. Examples of vendors who offer claims processing systems are listed in Figure 6.9.

Many of the available systems have origins in indemnity-based products and have been adapted to a managed care environment. A few products were designed specifically for HMOs or PPOs and serve the needs of specialized organizations quite well. Most vendors, however, are struggling to keep pace with a

Advanta (previously AIH)
Computer Sciences Corporation (CSC)
Electronic Data Systems - Health Care Division (EDS)
Erisco
GTE
Health System Integration, Inc. (HSII)
Health Systems Design Corp (HSD)
Reilly Dike Dosher Corporation (RDD)
RIMS

Figure 6.9   *Examples of Vendors of Claims Processing Systems*

rapidly changing marketplace. Point-of-service (POS) plans, for example, are becoming increasingly popular with employers attempting to control costs without limiting employees' choices of physicians. POS plans offer members the option of obtaining care through an HMO, a PPO, or an independent provider. POS plans maintain different benefits, copayments, and deductibles for members, depending on where in the system they receive care.

Systems supporting POS plans must support HMO functionality (e.g., capitation and risk pools), PPO functionality (e.g., claims repricing based on global fees or discount fee for service), and regular fee for service. As may be inferred, POS plans present a formidable challenge to vendors attempting to address the myriad possibilities that may be encountered.

In addition to adjudicating claims and calculating reimbursements, managed care systems must support a range of other functions requiring some level of support is in Figure 6.10.

Marketing and Sales Support	• Rate management/actuarial services • Contract management • Account management • Account analysis
Membership Accounting	• Government accounts (Medicare, Medicaid, Champus, FEP) • Individual coverage - COBRA, direct pay, pension plan • Group billing - benefits administration, eligibility determination
Service Delivery and Utilization Management	• Performance statistics • UM support • UM communication • Point-of-service intervention - eligibility, protocols, case management
Claims Payment and Prospective Reimbursement Processing	• Capitation payments • Claims (in network and out of network) • Encounters
Management Control and Reporting	• Membership analysis • Utilization rates • Quality indicators • Financial reporting • Regulatory reports

Figure 6.10   *Health Plan Core Functions*

Member/Consumer Services

From a member's or consumer's perspective, managed care technology may mean the system that he or she can load onto a home computer for educational purposes or facilitation of some type of electronic link with a provider. A number of strategies are emerging in this area that offer significant opportunities to reduce costs and increase quality in the care-delivery process. A few areas are:

- *Demand Management.* Most efforts today to control health care costs focus on increasing the efficiency of health care delivery. Demand management, on the other hand, focuses on reducing *demand* for health care services altogether. Demand management addresses health promotion, disease prevention, and consumer education. Demand management offers enormous opportunities for cost reduction by addressing the approximately 70 percent of health care dollars spent on preventable illness.

- *Member Education (Health Promotion).* Member education, or health promotion, is one aspect of demand management. Examples include mass mailings of wellness publications to all members or targeted mailings to certain high-risk or diagnosis-related populations. Member education also includes automated health reference guides that may be purchased for home use, such as A.D.A.M., Body Works, Family Health Tracker, Family Pharmacist, HealthDesk, Mayo Clinic Series, Medical Matters, The Complete Guide to Prescription and Non-Prescription Drugs, The Complete Guide to Symptoms, Illness and Surgery, The Doctor's Book of Home Remedies, The Family Doctor, and The Personal Physician.

  Member education techniques are also being extended to other areas, including preoperative and postoperative education for specific procedures. Educating patients before and after surgery can speed the recovery process and reduce the occurrence of readmission.

■ *Triage Systems.* Triage is also an aspect of demand management. Triage systems are generally used at a call-in desk for a health plan. The software guides the call taker through a list of questions and responses based on the caller's supplied information. The software helps in determining the urgency of care as well as the directing of care. Examples include Informed Access and Access Health Marketing. These vendors will license the software or provide a call-center service.

■ *Home Monitoring.* Home monitoring enables a member's health to be tracked by the health care system while the patient remains at home. This capability minimizes stress on the member while reducing the need for more costly face-to-face monitoring. Currently, home-based health care represents just 3 percent of health care spending nationwide, but the Congressional Budget Office predicts that amount will quadruple by the year 2000. This expansion of home health care services will drive the development of systems that make it possible to monitor patients in their own homes.

An example of home monitoring technology, piloted in Indianapolis in early 1995 by Quantum Health Resources, supports home-based treatment of hemophilia patients. With the software, patients keep logs of their daily infusion treatments and send the records via modem to Quantum for review. The software was developed by HealthDesk Corporation and can be expanded to support other home-based treatments such as high-risk pregnancies, diabetes, pneumonia, cancer, cystic fibrosis, and chronic heart conditions. The software also supports educational programs to provide a comprehensive approach to treatment of specific diseases.

- *Patient Satisfaction Surveys.* Patient satisfaction surveys attempt to measure quality of life factors as indicators of clinical outcomes. Examples of survey forms include the RAND 36-Item Health Survey. Companies like Velocity Healthcare Informatics provide systems or services that automate the administration, collection, and analysis of patient satisfaction surveys.

Meeting Employer Needs

Technology supporting employer needs surrounds the exchange of information between employers and health plans. This includes enrollment information from employers and outcomes information from the health plan.

- *Enrollment.* Employers and payers are working to refine the exchange of enrollment information. The value of automating this information is in maintaining an up-to-date membership database, combined with automated eligibility, in order to provide a mechanism for providers to handle patient accounts more effectively. Other savings can be attributed to the reduction of manual effort required to enter enrollment information into the system. Many vendors listed in Figure 6.9 are enhancing their systems to accept electronic enrollment transactions.

- *HEDIS Reporting.* HEDIS (Health Plan and Employer Data Information Set) is a set of performance measures designed to standardize the way health plans report data to employers. HEDIS focuses on four major performance areas: quality, access and patient satisfaction, membership and utilization, and finance. HEDIS was originally organized in late 1989 by The HMO Group, a national coalition of group and staff model HMOs. The New England HEDIS Coalition is a group of employers and health plans who are collaborating to develop a strategy for implementing HEDIS from both the health plans and employer perspectives.

Quality indicators includes childhood immunization rates, cholesterol screening, mammography rates, and other indicators. Membership and utilization includes enrollment and disenrollment statistics broken out by age and sex as well as measures such as hospital discharge rates and service rates. Patient satisfaction measures the members' satisfaction within their plans, procedure frequency rates, ambulatory-care visit rates, and mental health Finance focuses on information used to compile rates. This includes per-member, per-month revenue requirements, major cost components of rates, and rate trends.

HEDIS and HEDIS-like reporting capabilities are becoming increasingly important for health plans as buyers of health care begin to purchase based on standardized measures. Technology is quickly becoming a requirement for extracting HEDIS and other outcome information from existing or new information systems.

■ *Access to health plan or third-party administrator (TPA) information.* Beyond outcome and performance measures, employers may also want access to other information for specific purposes. For example, they may want access to targeted information in order to identify high-risk work areas. Additionally, self-funded employers need access to a wide range of information to support cost-saving and quality initiatives. This type of ad hoc information can be provided through core systems as long as the systems are flexible and easy to modify.

Managing Primary and Specialty Care

A number of technologies support management of primary care and specialist networks. These technologies include:

- *Credentialing Systems.* Credentialing refers to obtaining and reviewing the documentation of professional providers. Such documentation includes licensure, certifications, insurance, evidence of malpractice insurance, malpractice history, and so on. The credentialing process generally includes both reviewing information submitted by the provider as well as verification that the information is correct and complete. A credentialing system tracks provider credentials and generates notices when providers must be recredentialed. In general, a credentialing system is a standard requirement for health plans and has few strategic implications. Many existing claims processing systems support provider credentialing.

- *Provider Profiling.* Provider profiling is essential in a closed-panel plan supporting the need to identify high-cost providers. Plan medical directors use the information as a means of modifying behavior or for some level of corrective action. The value of provider profiling can be measured against the ability to lower the costs associated with high-cost providers in the network.

In addition to technologies for managing provider networks, other technologies such as health information networks and computer-based patient record systems directly support providers and also offer strategic advantages for the health plan. A few of the functions where automation supports more efficient processes or new capabilities include:

- Electronic eligibility and benefits inquiry
- Provider directory
- Electronic referrals and authorizations
- Electronic claims processing and reimbursement
- Enterprise scheduling
- Clinical guidelines

Managing the Delivery Network

One of the ways managed care organizations control costs is by defining in advance how a facility will be reimbursed for specific services. Managed care organizations attempt to build into the reimbursement methodology incentives for reducing utilization without compromising quality. This becomes a balancing act as managed care organizations attempt to set up arrangements that meet their needs and also are acceptable to the hospital or delivery network. The result may be a complex web of procedural and reimbursement guidelines that are difficult to map against the stream of claims generated by the facility.

Hospital billing systems cannot accommodate these complex reimbursement arrangements, and administrators are forced to calculate the correct reimbursement manually or simply trust the payer to calculate it for them. As the volume of claims priced under contractual agreements increases, however, manual intervention becomes increasingly cumbersome and ineffective. Administrators may employ spreadsheets or other tools to help, but these types of solutions are only temporary and cannot meet expanding needs.

The solution is a contract management system that calculates expected reimbursement based on the contract rules. Contract management systems support a variety of reimbursement arrangements, including:

- Fee for service
- Discounted fee for service
- Diagnosis-Related Groups (DRGs)
- Global fees
- Per diem rates
- Capitation

Capitation support includes the ability to reconcile capitation payments, track incurred but not reported (IBNR) costs, and manage risk pools. Contract management systems also support combinations of these arrangements based on a service. For example, a contract management system may have to support a fixed reimbursement for a procedure plus a diminishing per diem amount for each day after, say, the third day in the hospital.

Contract management products often include other features such as decision support, modeling and forecasting, cost reporting, and contract compliance tracking.

The focus of contract management systems is to maximize revenues for the facility by ensuring that services are reimbursed according to contractual terms. Contract management systems are sound investments for facilities that have a number of contractual relationships with managed care organizations. Numerous anecdotal stories attest to recovered revenues in the millions of dollars and systems paying for themselves in a few months.

While contract management systems clearly help administrators maximize revenues, they do not support enhanced quality of care or cost-reduction initiatives. Consequently, a contract management system represents more of a short-term tactical solution rather than a long-term strategic initiative.

In addition to contract management, a range of other technologies are required to support managed care initiatives within the delivery system, such as:

- Precertification/assignment of length of stay (LOS)

- Clinical guidelines/critical pathways

- Case management/large case management

- Outcomes reporting

- Acuity measures

- Severity adjusting

- Carve-outs/centers of excellence

- Utilization management

- Enterprise scheduling
- Master Person Index
- Computerized Patient Record systems
- Electronic data interchange

Master Person Index (MPI)[4]

In our changing health care industry, the criticality of an MPI solution for integrated delivery systems is increasing as acquisitions continue and health systems expand. This criticality was underscored by the American Health Information Management Association[5] (AHIMA) in its April 1994 position statement on managing health information in facility mergers and acquisitions. In this document AHIMA stated, "To ensure availability of health information to all legitimate users, patient records should be consolidated or linked in the master patient index." The statement goes on to discuss the role of the MPI for merged facilities and possible options for linking patient records.

The AHIMA position reflects the information technology void that is formed when health care organizations form alliances or merge. The first step in filling this void is to build an MPI system that addresses the needs of the integrated delivery system (IDS). However, the process of building an MPI can be complicated, and issues beyond the control of the CIO will impact the final outcome. Issues that affect the optimal solution include organization size and composition, types of relationships between entities, legacy systems, and the competitive environment in the local marketplace.

Person versus Patient

The health care system as a whole is shifting away from encounter-based care to covered lives. Similarly, the focus of the MPI within an integrated delivery system will likewise shift away from a patient focus toward a broader member or person focus. To reflect this shift, it may be appropriate to modify the terminology so that the master *patient* index becomes the master *person* index. This broader definition more accurately reflects the growing needs of health systems as they begin to track wellness as a part of their comprehensive care process.

Value of the Master Person Index

Historically the role of the master patient index has been to assist admitting or registration personnel in locating prior visit information and to support the integration of patient information within a facility. The challenge for the facility administrator attempting to link to existing patient records may have involved an inpatient system, an outpatient system, and even an emergency department system, all of which could have maintained their own patient numbering schemes. An MPI could facilitate the process of locating existing patient information, regardless of where it was stored, reducing some of the administrative burden associated with the admitting or registration process.

A primary goal of the MPI was to ensure that patient demographic information, once entered into the system, was consistent across disparate systems and was available for subsequent encounters. Another goal was to ensure that all electronically stored information about a patient was linked and available to administrators for billing and management purposes. To support these goals, the MPI had to provide the ability to locate and access patient information from disparate systems, given that the information provided to the operator may not exactly have matched the information stored in the system.

To find and link records based on imprecise information, an MPI requires an algorithm for identifying possible matches of candidate records. Records could be flagged based on close matches of simple demographic information such as Social Security number, name, age, height, weight, sex, and so on, allowing that attributes such as the Social Security number could be falsi-fied, surnames could be spelled differently or changed, and nicknames could be used in place of first names. Given the pos-sibilities, some MPI systems assigned a probability that a se-lected record was a match and allowed the operator to make the final determination.

Many organizations found that the best strategy for ad-dressing their needs was to implement a common admitting or registration system that had MPI functionality built into it. Using this strategy, the common admitting or registration sys-tem tracked the unique identifiers for each application that had its own internal patient demographic information and patient identification schemes. The common admitting or registration system then became the single point of entry and control mech-anism for patient identification and demographic information for the facility.

The single-hospital MPI model clearly meets the needs of hospital administrators attempting to access patient records contained in one or more disparate applications within a hospi-tal. However, problems that the MPI addresses at the hospital level are again being encountered at the integrated delivery sys-tem level except on a much larger scale. As health care organi-zations merge to form integrated delivery systems, many are finding that they are again searching for ways to link records contained in disparate computer systems. Only this time the number of systems may be much larger, and the distance be-tween systems may be much greater.

The driver behind the need to link these systems is the same as that behind the formation of integrated delivery sys-tems themselves: managed care. To effectively compete in a managed care environment, a health system must control costs and manage care across the continuum of care. It is fundamen-tal to this process that administrators have the ability to track a patient across multiple facilities through multiple episodes of care. For a health system that has incurred risk for a member, it is imperative that utilization is closely managed and that any information already in the system (such as lab or radiology results or medication information) be cataloged to reduce costly duplication of effort or wasted resources. For providers delivering care under contracted arrangements (per diem, discounted fee for service, etc.), patients must be closely tracked across multiple entities to ensure adherence to the contracts and to support utilization management requirements.

It is clear that integrated delivery systems are placing new demands on the MPI. What is not clear, however, is how to address the need for an MPI for a multifacility, multiservice organization. Additionally, questions arise as to the impact of a universal patient identification system and the role of an MPI in community, regional, and national health care information networks. CIOs must sort through these issues in order to determine the most appropriate approach for their organization.

Profile of a Master Person Index

In developing a strategy for an integrated delivery system MPI, CIOs will encounter several options. The viability and practicality of each option depend on the unique environment of the IDS. Three fundamental options follow.

Option 1: Extend the Registration System

The first option for addressing the needs of an integrated delivery system is to extrapolate the approach taken inside the hospital—that is, implement a single registration system for the enterprise. In this solution, MPI functionality is imbedded in the common registration system, and patient identification numbers are assigned according to the scheme used by the common system. This solution, shown in Figure 6.11, is simple and relatively straightforward.

This solution may work best for a smaller integrated delivery system that will likely maintain a compact profile. For larger health systems, however, this solution becomes more complex. Registration systems designed for single facilities may

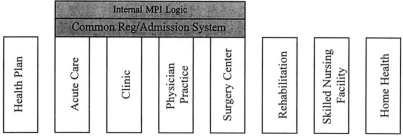

Figure 6.11 *Extended Registration System*

reach technical limitations when extended too far. Additionally, the economics of replacing a number of registration systems may be questionable depending on current functionality, the potential organizational impact of a system conversion, and budget constraints and priorities.

Option 2: Link Registration Systems through an Enterprise MPI

A second option is to maintain existing registration systems and link them via a master person index. In this solution the MPI acts as an umbrella application that links registration systems from various facilities or departments within the integrated delivery system. An indexing system is used for the master file, and individual records contain pointers to patient records in various applications within the integrated delivery system. The pointers provide the access paths to patient records (from individual health care organizations) and member records (from a health plan). The master file indexing system may be internal to the MPI or based on an enterprisewide identification scheme adopted by the IDS. Individual organizations or departments may continue to use their existing system and patient identification schemes.

Procedurally, prior to or during admission or registration, the admitting or registration clerk would enter basic demographic information about the patient into the MPI application. Information could be entered manually or via a smart card.

When information is unreliable, such as for a manual data entry where a patient's identification number is unavailable, a list of probable matches may be displayed. The clerk can be prompted to ask questions to narrow the list and confirm that the correct patient record is selected. This solution is shown in Figure 6.12.

Once the correct MPI record is identified, the clerk can access the information necessary to register the patient. An integrated MPI application may have the ability to download identification information directly to the admission or registration system. If no prior record exists or if existing information is outdated, the MPI may download the necessary demographic and insurance information to the admission or registration system.

The advantage of this solution is that it supports a growth strategy for integrated delivery systems. Existing admission or registration systems do not have to be converted, and existing patient identification schemes do not have to be changed. Further, the IDS can support loosely affiliated organizations under the same MPI umbrella. These advantages can enable an IDS to focus resources on expanding the service network rather than on retrofitting IDS facilities and departments.

The disadvantage of this strategy is that the MPI application is not fundamentally integrated. An effort is required to

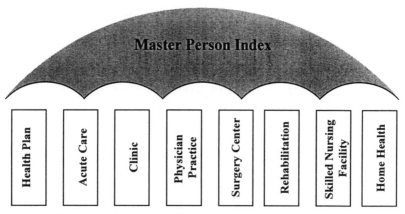

Figure 6.12 *Link Registration Systems*

facilitate transmission of basic demographic and insurance information from the MPI application to each of the subordinate admission or registration systems. If the MPI is not integrated with existing admission or registration systems, the user may have to deal with two different user interfaces, or even two different terminals, and be faced with the task of manually transcribing information from the MPI application to the admission or registration system.

Option 3: Status Quo—Operate without an MPI

A third option is to continue operations without an MPI. In this strategy, administrators have the option of providing clerks with the ability to access multiple admission or registration systems and effectively do the MPI search manually or simply allow multiple records to accumulate within the IDS. If most of the organization's revenue is derived from fee-for-service arrangements or if the IDS is relatively small, this strategy works by minimizing capital investment in new applications. Manual procedures may be implemented to enhance efficiency, and batch processes can be written to identify probabilistic matches and link records within one or more databases. In effect, procedures and periodic batch processes can offset the negative effects of not having integrated access to all patient records within an IDS as long as the IDS is small and penetration of managed care in the community is limited. This solution is shown in Figure 6.13.

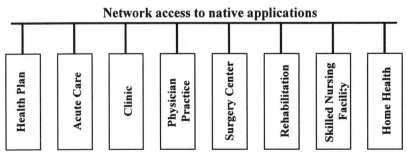

Figure 6.13 *Operate without an MPI*

State of the Market

The demand for enterprisewide MPI systems will continue to grow as the health care industry continues its path of affiliations, mergers, and acquisitions. Vendors are reacting to the demand and are offering solutions that link information from a variety of sources within an integrated delivery system. As of early 1995, Shared Medical Systems, Corporation (SMS) was offering Enterprise Access Directory (EAD) as an enterprise solution; Ameritech Health Connections was building an MPI into its health information network software; IDX was developing the Enterprise Patient Management System (EPMS) for its solution set; and Epic Systems, Corporation offered MPI functionality through its enterprise scheduling module. Additionally, vendors such as HBOC/First Data, who offer computer-based patient record (CPR) solutions, were expanding their scope to meet the needs of the enterprise rather than just a single facility. For these expanded CPR solutions an IDS MPI is an inherent component of the overall product.

The MPI, however, should not be viewed as the final solution. An MPI is only the first critical step in linking information between disparate systems within an IDS. Although an MPI can be viewed as an essential step toward a CPR, an MPI cannot offer much of the functionality required of a CPR by an IDS, such as the ability to measure performance or outcomes. The role of an MPI within an IDS is very definite and narrowly defined. This role, however, is a foundation block that is essential to a long-term IDS information integration strategy.

CIOs revising their strategic information systems plans should give consideration to the role of an MPI in their technology strategy. The urgency of an MPI depends on a number of conditions, including the current systems environment, strategic business goals, alliances, planned mergers, the local market, and so on. The pace for implementing an MPI should be driven by the value it offers the organization, and the value of an MPI is based on the IDS's ability to leverage the tool to enhance the quality of care, control costs, and gain a competitive advantage in the marketplace.

Enterprise Scheduling[6]

Administrators are finding that one of the keys to unlocking additional advantages of a larger health system is through enterprise scheduling capabilities. Enterprise scheduling is an essential element for bringing disparate organizations together and optimizing resources within an IDS. Enterprise scheduling capabilities also support quality initiatives aimed at member access and patient satisfaction. Quality measures such as patient satisfaction are becoming increasingly important as the Health Plan Employer Data and Information Set is refined and employers begin to rely on HEDIS measures for selecting health plans.

Unfortunately, the solution to enterprise scheduling is not necessarily easy, and administrators implementing enterprise scheduling systems may have to deal with multiple facilities and multiple legacy scheduling systems. Depending on the environment, administrators may face a number of challenges in developing a solution.

Profile of Enterprise Scheduling Systems

A scheduling system controls the use of services or limited-access resources such as magnetic resonance imaging (MRI) equipment. Depending on the type of service, scheduling systems may be simple or complex. A surgery center, for example, requires the ability to block and schedule rooms based on predefined requirements. Figure 6.14 illustrates how a surgery center allocates rooms for procedures based on specialty. In this case, specialists from different groups know when they may schedule their patients for procedures in the surgery center. If

	OR #1	OR #2	OR #3	OR #4	OR #5	OR #6	OR #7
Monday	GEN	ORTHO	GEN	CARDIAC	PEDS	URO PEDS	URO
				CARDIAC	PEDS	ORAL	OPTH
Tuesday	GEN	ORTHO	URO	CARDIAC	GYN	URO	OPTH
			ORTHO	CARDIAC	GYN	URO	OPTH
Wednesday	GEN	ORTHO	VASC	NEURO	GYN	URO	PLASTIC
			VASC	NEURO		GEN	PLASTIC

Figure 6.14   *Block Schedule for a Surgery Center*

they do not confirm the room at least 24 hours in advance, for example, the room may be released for rescheduling.

Scheduling systems automate many of the administrative-intensive tasks behind scheduling a service or resource. Capabilities of a typical scheduling system include

- Conflict checking

- Searching for available slots

- Scheduling multiple resources (e.g., physician, room, equipment, technician)

- Printing reminders, cancellation notices, no-show notices

- Maintaining a wait list

- Generating medical record chart pull

- Scheduling recurring or cyclical appointments

- Generating resource utilization reports

Scheduling systems, in general, were developed to serve niche markets and have strengths and weaknesses based on their origins. Scheduling systems originally developed for inpatient facilities may be strong in their ability to support resource scheduling but may be weak in their ability to support outpatient facility needs. Conversely, scheduling systems developed for outpatient environments may be strong in their ability to support scheduling of services such as office visits but may lack an ability to support resource scheduling for MRI equipment.

Additionally, like other technologies in the health care industry, most scheduling systems were originally developed with a single facility in mind. These systems were not designed to integrate or coordinate with other scheduling systems. The result is that administrators are faced with the challenge of developing a solution palatable to end users as well as acceptable to budget hawks in the finance department.

Enterprise Scheduling Systems

Enterprise scheduling systems enable physician groups, hospitals, and other facilities within an enterprise to act as a single organization and easily schedule needed services or resources, regardless of where they are in the enterprise. A strategy for achieving this capability is to replace existing scheduling systems with a single enterprisewide scheduling system. In this strategy, separate facilities access a single centralized scheduling system to meet their individual needs. Many of the products on the market today allow the scheduling function to be centralized or decentralized. In a decentralized approach, the products allow administrators to control the latitude administrative staffs have in scheduling other facilities' resources. Some of the benefits of an enterprise scheduling system are listed in Figure 6.15.

A number of vendors are beginning to offer enterprise scheduling solutions that support this strategy. Vendors that provide these solutions generally have enhanced or rewritten niche products to meet a broader range of needs. Other vendors are leveraging existing outpatient scheduling products to meet the needs of larger integrated delivery systems.

- Better patient flow throughout organization
- Increased productivity with time efficiencies for physician office and ancillary staff
- Optimized utilization of all resources, providers, staff, space, and equipment
- Better communication between departments
- Increased and consistent communication to patients regarding expectations
- Management reporting at multiple levels of detail
- Improved patient satisfaction
- Better relations with physicians

Figure 6.15   *Value of Enterprise Scheduling*

An enterprise scheduling strategy does provide a few challenges for administrators. First, it requires that a number of operation and control issues be addressed. Most departments are reluctant to allow staff from other facilities to schedule appointments in their facility or department. These types of control issues, if not resolved, can hamper the strategy. Second, replacement of legacy scheduling systems may be required. And administrators face an uphill battle if the new system does not support the niche needs of a facility as well as the existing system. Third, the new system will have to be linked to an existing hospital information system. Scheduling packages must be able to retrieve demographic information to support basic scheduling functions.

Linking Systems

A key element of an enterprise scheduling strategy is in linking the scheduling system to legacy systems. This effort is required to maximize the functionality available in niche products. The challenge behind this effort is to develop the links between systems in a way that supports a full range of functionality and data integrity.

This type of integration effort is currently being pursued by St. Agnes Hospital in Fresno, California. St. Agnes uses HBOC's Star application set in the hospital and has linked the health information system to Enterprise Systems' (ESI) scheduling application. In this setup requests for appointments are called into a centralized scheduling pool where operators schedule the procedures on the ESI system. St. Agnes uses CL7 scripting language from Century Analysis (CAI) to automatically retrieve demographic information from the Star system and populate fields on the ESI scheduling screens. Scheduling information is then routed through the interface engine (CAI's Transaction Distribution Manager) and back to the Star system. Scheduling information is maintained on the Star system to provide access to hospital-based users. Additionally, St. Agnes uses the Star scheduling module for scheduling hospital-based resources such as radiology procedures.

One reason St. Agnes selected this strategy was to take advantage of a linkage between ESI's enterprise scheduling module and ESI's NOVA materials management module. With this link, materials are automatically ordered based on the scheduled procedure. This illustrates some of the advantages that can be gained when administrators look beyond traditional boundaries while assessing the value of a technology.

Other linkages are also possible. Enterprisewide scheduling systems may be interfaced to transportation systems. Additionally, many tests and procedures that are scheduled require orders to be placed through the order management system. Scheduling systems may be linked to order management systems to support this type of functionality. Future integration may be appropriate with staff allocation systems to calculate staffing based on expected resource utilization.

HL7

Today linking scheduling systems together or with other applications can be a challenging task. However, this will change as standards for scheduling systems are developed. Health Level Seven (HL7) is currently in the process of drafting an enterprise scheduling standard. This standard defines the format and content of messages for communicating scheduling events. The draft standard outlines four categories of applications as related to a scheduling event: a placer application, a filler application, a querying application, and an auxiliary application.

> A placer application requests the booking, modification, cancellation, etc., of a scheduled activity for a service or resource. . . . A filler application . . . is one that 'owns' one or more schedules for one or more services or resources. . . . A querying application . . . is only concerned with gathering information about a particular schedule. . . . An auxiliary application passively collects information by receiving unsolicited updates from a filler application.

The relationship between these applications is shown in Figure 6.16.

Although this standard will not be official for a while, it is important to recognize its impact. The standard provides an avenue for selecting scheduling products based on the ability to

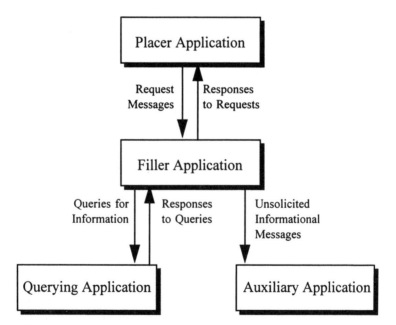

Figure 6.16 *Application Role Messaging Relationships (HL7)*

serve niche needs while still leveraging the benefits of information sharing.

State of the Market

In addition to vendors offering enterprise scheduling solutions, some traditional health information systems vendors are recognizing the need to offer enterprisewide scheduling systems as integrated components of their products. Additionally, a few vendors of physician practice management have scheduling modules that are integrated with their products.

Universal Interface Engines[7]

The advent of mixed-platform and vendor information services shops has resulted in the issues of multiple user interfaces, redundant data entry, and multiple occurrences of the same data elements. Having multiple entry points and storage locations for the same data elements, in turn, leads to complex and resource-consuming data integrity problems. In the past, health care administrators addressed the data integrity problems by controlling the number of manual entry points and building custom interfaces to pass data between applications. Building point-to-point interfaces between a small number of applications is a reasonable approach for this problem; however, as the number of niche applications increases, the network becomes increasingly complex and difficult to maintain.

Value of a Universal Interface Engine

Figure 6.17 illustrates the complexity involved with interfacing 6 applications in a worst-case scenario in which each application must interface with each of the 5 remaining applications. As this example shows, there are 30 point-to-point interfaces

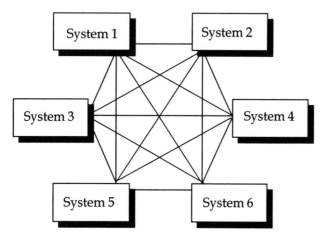

Total Number of Interfaces = n(n-1)

Figure 6.17   *Point-to-Point Interfaces*

$(6 \times (6 - 1) = 30)$. System 1 to System 2 is one interface, System 2 to System 1 is a second interface, and so forth.

In some cases the cost of building new custom interfaces for replacement of one system could exceed the cost of the system. As can be deduced from the figure, changing one system in this worst-case scenario requires modification or rewriting of 10 interfaces. Because costs may range from $10,000 to $100,000 per interface, the cost of completely integrating a new system into the environment becomes prohibitive.

To address cost issues related to development and maintenance of point-to-point interfaces within a diverse systems environment, administrators now have the option of employing a universal interface engine. Universal interface engines perform the protocol translation for the individual applications and thus reduce the need to develop customized applications programming interfaces (APIs). Although the individual applications must be able to generate or receive interface messages, they no longer must reformat messages or maintain routing information for each message type. Figure 6.18 illustrates the concept of an interface engine.

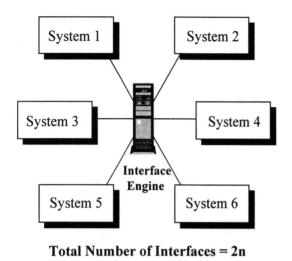

Total Number of Interfaces = 2n

Figure 6.18 *Employing an Interface Engine*

As this exhibit shows, there are 12 interfaces ($2 \times 6 = 12$) in this example, and only two must be modified when one system is replaced. Although the cost of the interface engine is a factor, using an interface engine to link different systems can reduce the costs of interfacing disparate systems by up to 90 percent.

Profile of a Universal Interface Engine

An interface engine has both hardware and software components. The hardware may range from a high-end server platform, such as IBM's RS/6000 running AIX or a low-end Intel-based PC running either DOS or OS/2. The software generally consists of a high-performance third generation language, such as C, and an internal database management system for storing routing and message formatting information. Interface engines use a three-step process for controlling interface transactions:

- The interface engine receives application-generated messages in native format off the network or from a direct physical connection.

■ The interface engine then reformats the messages based on scripting information stored in its internal database. The engine maintains scripting information for every message type that it is required to handle.

■ Finally, the interface engine retransmits the messages back to the appropriate destinations. The destination information is also maintained in the scripts.

In addition to saving costs and time on critical projects, interface engines enable health care providers to expand their scope and interface applications they otherwise might not have. These advantages can be significant for health care institutions that have been struggling with data integrity problems and heavy interface development workloads.

Strategically, use of these products positions health care institutions for future growth and flexibility. The cost of replacing or adding new systems will no longer be prohibitive, and health care professionals will no longer have to limit their choice of viable clinical applications based solely on what will or will not fit into the existing systems environment.

Summary

The technologies profiled in this chapter support emerging trends and growing needs in the health care marketplace. These technologies are significantly different from those traditionally addressed in strategic information systems plans of just a few years ago. Strategic information plans of yesterday addressed the needs of individual departments and gave little consideration to the value of shared technology. Today's plans should no longer focus solely on individual departments but on the entire health system. This type of focus is required to enable a competitive advantage in a market where buyers are focusing on cost, quality, and access.

In addition, health care organizations can no longer afford to view information technology as simply a support function. Technology must be applied in a strategic manner providing the ability to reengineer existing processing and to develop new products and services. Applying technology in this type of strategic manner will greatly leverage potential benefits and provide the competitive advantage needed to survive in a rapidly changing marketplace.

Notes

1. Adapted from original publication in *Healthcare Informatics*, February 1994.

2. News 33/400 March 1992.

3. Workgroup on Electronic Data Interchange, Financial Implications Subcommittee, Technical Advisory Group, 1993.

4. Adapted from original publication in *Healthcare Informatics*, November 1994.

5. American Health Information Management Association in their April 1994 position statement.

6. Adapted from original publication in *Healthcare Informatics*, February 1995.

7. Adapted from original publication in *Healthcare Informatics*, July 1993.

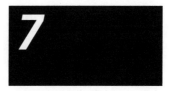

7

The People Part

Overview

Information systems departments within the health care industry must align their organizational model(s) with those structures needed to support the business enterprise they service. Integrated health information networks (HINs), managed care, and the merger-affiliation mania—all discussed earlier in this book—require information systems managers to reshape their departments to create synergy with the institution's business mission.

Technology deployment is predicated on people. People, not technology, will make the most difference in an information services department's success. Roles and responsibilities must be clearly articulated so information systems professionals can deliver necessary functionality to the organization. The organization chart is the first place people look to understand what is expected of them.

So what organizational factors should the health care CIO consider in facing these constantly changing priorities and demands? How does he allocate resources among competing initiatives? How does she create an organization that can meet the sweeping agenda for new systems, new capabilities, and new levels of performance?

This chapter will examine how information services departments should be positioned, organized, and led to be able to support the strategic agenda emerging within the health care industry. It is within the context of these conditions that the future view of the new information technology (IT) organization must be developed. This chapter will discuss organizational strategies for addressing the following issues:

- Dynamics of governance and expectations management

- Organizational responsiveness and flexibility

- Organizational structures and models

- Organizational tools necessary to deliver IT services and

- CIO's role in effecting transition to the future-state IT organization

Governance

As the health care enterprise evolves, traditional methods for selecting information systems initiatives will also need to change. The first step is to craft a plan that will be aligned with the enterprisewide strategic vision. The plan will need to evolve, sometimes rather quickly, as the enterprise implements the HIN strategic agenda. Although the strategic goals may not change significantly, the tactics by which the strategies are achieved will be in constant flux. Assumptions that drove the information systems (IS) strategic plan will be challenged; changing alliances between entities in the HIN will change the scope and character of the needs for information systems; the cast of leaders will change as well.

Along with this will come an entirely new set of clients, ranging from the primary-care physician practice leader to the CEO of the HIN's insurance entity. Each client organization brings its own decision-making processes, resource allocation perspectives, and organizational cultures to the discussions about how best to implement the IS strategic agenda. Each brings a unique view of the role of information systems in transforming the enterprise.

In this section we explore techniques by which the CIO can build an effective governance process to guide the IS organization during implementation of the IS strategic plan while dealing with:

- Concurrent enterprise initiatives that create conflicting IS objectives—sometimes not discovered until the initiative is well underway

- Communications about changing tactics that are never fast enough, complete enough, or reliable enough

- Intense competition for talented people and

- Almost continuous change in the enterprisewide organization structures, leadership, and affiliations.

Dynamics of Governance

Foundations for governance are created during the IS strategic planning process. As the planning process builds a composite view of enterprise needs, it also builds a cadre of knowledgeable people who understand the plan's premise, the strategic underpinnings, and the dynamics of the planning process itself. The plan defines the governance structures, that is, the principles, standards, and procedures by which the enterprise will implement the strategic plan. The plan represents the enterprise's best view of its needs and strategies for addressing those needs as understood at that point in time.

Yet, as we have discussed earlier, the evolving nature of the HIN will result in the need for constant shifts and adjustments to the plan. In the past this could be accommodated through a periodic review or update of the IS strategic plan. In the future, however, this will need to become a much more dynamic process that occurs almost constantly. The plan will be subjected to reality testing, to relevancy tests, and to financial viability tests at every step of implementation. To make this viable, there will be a critical need for governance processes that can quickly and accurately:

- Detect shifts in the environment

- Detect shifts in HIN goals as they emerge from the reengineering initiatives and evolving affiliations or mergers

- Make very responsive decisions about the IS priorities, that is, what to start, what to stop, what to change, and how to allocate resources.

To achieve this level of agility, the same people who participated in the initial IS strategic planning process need to drive the governance processes. Who are they? In most HINs they are the organizational stakeholders, so it will be important to keep adjusting the governance membership as the enterprise changes structure and leadership. In addition, it will be important to include stakeholders who technically are not part of the enterprise but have a strategic role in attainment of the enterprise's objectives (e.g., alliance partners). The CIO's challenge will be to find ways to entice them into participating in the governance process.

Governance Models

While governance models are still evolving in the HIN arena, certain characteristics are emerging:

- Membership crosses organizational boundaries.

- The emphasis is on delivering seamless capabilities everywhere.

- Every initiative is tested for strategic relevance repeatedly.

- Knowledge development is an ongoing process.

Ideally, the governance organization's structure should be closely aligned with that of the enterprise. We suggest that the CIO look at these three basic models as a starting point for designing his own model:

- *Centralized Strategic Control with Decentralized Execution.* In this approach a centralized (enterprisewide) group has the responsibility to ensure that the IS plan stays aligned with the enterprise business strategies and tactics. This may be a subcommittee of the enterprisewide strategic business planning committee or a subgroup of the enterprise executive management team. Although the IS strategic planning committee might continue to function in this role, we believe the governance process must be driven by those with the organizational power to make the governance process legitimate. Each entity in the enterprise should also have a governance group, made up of the local stakeholders, that guides the local execution of the enterprisewide strategies and provides input to the centralized group on needs and priorities based on their local perspective of the enterprise goals.

■ *Centralized Strategic Control and Execution.* This approach also relies on a centralized enterprisewide group to ensure the ongoing alignment of the IS plan with the strategic business agenda. Two variations are likely to emerge:

    ■ Small group of key stakeholders make the key decisions, relying on a much larger group of stakeholders to advise them on specific issues and needs, or

    ■ Large group of key stakeholders make the key decisions, relying on each other to educate and advise.

■ *Completely Decentralized Control and Execution.* This approach uses existing governance groups in each of the enterprise entities that independently lobby the corporate CIO and executives for resources and priorities. The local entities may fully control the local resources as well as have access to independent resources. In this instance their interactions with the CIO are primarily about getting access to seamless enterprise capabilities.

Managing Expectations

As the tactics for reinventing the HIN become clearer, managing expectations at the governance level becomes a critical role for the CIO for a number of reasons.

- The needed applications are available in the marketplace but have not been designed for deployment in a large-scale, enterprisewide setting.

- The needed applications do not exist in the marketplace, require extensive development time and resources, and impose significant risk.

- The time frames for delivering system capabilities do not take into consideration the time needed to build the underlying infrastructure.

- Contention for key IS resources to guide or manage the projects becomes the limiting factor.

As the CIO formulates his own approach to these barriers, these perspectives may be helpful:

- It is crucial for the IS organization to actively participate in enterprisewide reengineering initiatives.

- The role of educator or subject-matter expert, needs to expand to include every member of the governance group.

- The newer stakeholders, especially direct-care providers, will inject dramatically higher expectations for responsiveness and speed, both in decision making and deployment.

- Bringing technology and resources from other industries may become a critical tactic for meeting the enterprise's objectives.

- Linking the IS organization to the governance organization must happen at levels below the CIO. Ideally, the key stakeholders within the IS organization should all take part in the governance process.

Organizational Responsiveness

As the pace of change accelerates throughout the enterprise, the CIO will find that established norms and performance standards for her organization are no longer acceptable. Projects that should take years to accomplish need to be done in months. Backlogs that are 12 to 24 months long need to be closed out in 6 months. Client department's expectations for technical competence include even less tolerance for uncertainty, and imprecision, and for technical risk. Communications within the CIO's organization, and with his clients, need to flow faster. Decisions need to be made today—not next week or next month.

From the client's perspective, IS responsiveness becomes a key factor in whether the client's own agenda for change can be accomplished. The CIO finds himself spending more and more time facilitating dialogue and decision making among his clients. The CIO spends more and more time dealing with interpersonal issues among team members. And she finds it essential to spend more time helping staff members understand the need to change priorities, shift resources, and change tactics week by week.

In this section we would like to explore the emerging performance measures and their implications for the CIO as the health information network matures.

The New Yardstick

Technical competence, prudent practices, thorough evaluations, conservative technologies—these have been traditional cornerstones of IS performance measures. Doing it right has been more important than doing it now. Or, conversely, doing it wrong has had stronger consequences than doing it late. Risk has always been something to avoid. Delivering technology has been the focus. Deriving benefits from technology has been the user's obligation, not the CIO's. The entire profession has measured itself using its own definition of competence.

So what's different now? Simply put, the established IS clients are finally demanding responsive services. As they reinvent their own business processes, they uncover key service attributes their clients expect. They discover new yardsticks. And they begin to reshape their own criteria for what constitutes effective services from the IS organization. Newer business partners bring their own expectations to the table as well—some driven by their past experience with IS, some with the levels of responsiveness they routinely have to provide in their own organizations.

Our message to the corporate CIO is this: *The yardstick will be changing very soon. It will assume that technical competence is fully present and deployed (no room at all for technical "softness"). We suggest you consider four performance measures from David Kantor of Goodmeasure that judge how "flexible, fast, friendly, and focused" the IS organization is, as viewed by its clients. Exceptional performance will only be acknowledged when it exceeds client expectations, not industry norms. Technologies will be assessed in terms of the benefits they deliver to the organization, as perceived by clients, not your staff. Finally, your clients are the ones wielding the yardstick, not you or your boss.*

Alignment to Meet "Client" Needs

At least four core issues will need to be addressed by the entire IS organization. They need to be explored in depth, ideally in a mission and values retreat format.

- Who are our clients?

- What are our obligations to our clients (our view)?

- What do they expect of us (their view)?

- How do our clients actually measure our performance (their yardstick)?

This is just the tip of the iceberg, yet it's a good place to begin these conversations. At some point it is helpful to invite the clients into the conversation as well. The synergy can be surprising.

Understanding how your clients are organized and how they deliver services to their own clients is also prerequisite to developing an effective service delivery strategy. Although technical service delivery mechanisms can be defined along functional lines (e.g., operations, development, database administration, etc.), client service mechanisms need to closely mirror the client organization's structure. Ideally, the IS organization should look and feel like an extension of the client's own organization. Ideally, your clients should participate in your IS performance appraisal processes. Ask your clients about this.

Access Considerations

Access and alignment go hand in hand. The intent of alignment is to facilitate client access to your services. In the past it was possible to implement procedures (obstacles) that effectively constrained access to IS resources. For some this was the only strategy available to deal with the flood of requests for help. In the coming environment it will still be important to carefully orchestrate the flow within the IS shop. However, what is needed by the clients is someone, a contact person, who:

- Is readily accessible

- Understands the client's business, services, and needs

- Can help the client clarify needs and turn them into requirements

- Can effectively represent client needs (an advocate) within the IS shop

- Can help the client learn how to take full advantage of technology

- Is committed to client success

Implications for the Information Systems Department

As the transformation continues, we believe that:

- Now is the right time to create a client-driven service organization. Even if you think you've got one, ask your clients. Listen openly and honestly to their reactions. Invite them to tell you about their yardsticks. As you acquire new clients, ask them, too.

- Continuing to build and strengthen the technical competence and capabilities of the organization is absolutely essential.

Organizational Structures

Information services departments do not vary substantially from institution to institution. Most departments have a position titled director of management information systems (MIS). A great number of facilities use the title chief information officer (CIO) to designate the top person in IS. Yet, most of these individuals are not members of the executive management team. It is not unusual to find at least one reporting layer between the CIO and chief executive. Most CIOs are not involved in decisions that dictate how their organization will function. Most CIOs do not control or even coordinate *all* aspects of information managed throughout the enterprise.

Organization structures for IS departments remain predominately hierarchical, self-contained, and multilayered. But many of these organizational characteristics are changing!

The Organization Chart

The current organization structure for many health care entities is challenging the historic rationale used to draft the organization chart. The information services department is now central to an organization's ability to deliver care to and conduct business with its patient or member population. The importance of the CIO has and will continue to grow. Since service delivery models, or organization charts, define how IS departments interact, communicate, and deliver services to their clients, we will look at the attributes and common characteristics of evolving organization structures.

The characteristics of the future state of health care, coupled with your organization's adoption of industry initiatives, will require executive management to assess which service delivery model will be most productive for a given enterprise. Management must determine how to draw the organizational chart to achieve maximum benefit from their IS resources.

Below are several outlined organizational models for IS departments today and in the future. For each alternative model, defining characteristics are identified to assist recognizing a model when it is being employed. Every model outlined, or a derivative thereof, is in use at one or more health care providers throughout the United States. Also, several parameters are outlined to assist the evaluation process when considering which model is most appropriate to serve as your baseline. Remember, these models are not an exhaustive list of choices, and a given model can serve as a guideline by which a tailored model could be developed specifically to an organization.

Prevailing Models

- *Outsource Model.* Shown in Figure 7.1, this organization alternative comes into focus when the prevalent requirement for IS is to rapidly implement responsive operational changes. Recognize that outsourcing arrangements transfer responsibility for service delivery

to an outs···   ···roup. Outsourcing firms tend to
be able to   ···e ···   eater sense of urgency when un-
dertakin···   ··· S implementation projects. With
downsiz···   ···-reduction pressures, outsourcing enab···   environment to generate predictable ope···   s and to shift away from full-time,
equivale···   staffing to service-level staffing.
Therefor···   ···ability and costing are no longer
predicate···   ··· presumption that a given position
must be f···   do the job, but rather on whether a
specific p···   ···r activity will be completed successfully unde···   ···ontrol of the outsourcer.

■ *Central Fl··· ···rarchical Model.* Shown in Figure 7.2,
this repres···   ···e traditional IS environment for many
health car···   ···nizations. There is usually a single
CIO, regar···   ···f the number of entities that comprise
the parent···   ···ization. In a multi-entity enterprise,
each entity···   ···ave an MIS director who directly reports to the···   ···porate CIO. There is a well-defined
chain of co···   ···nd. The sphere of influence for the
MIS directo···   is also well defined. It is common to
see a regional   ···a center supporting multiple facilities.
IS resource ···   ···cation and decision making occurs at
the top of the   ···organization structure. Finally, executive and line ···   ···agement look to a single point of contact for all IS ···   ···tters.

■ *Centralized O··· ···rsight Model.* Shown in Figure 7.3,
this organization has multiple entities with separate IS
departments under the umbrella of a corporate parent.
The corporate CIO *coordinates* IS services through
entity-specific MIS directors who hold independent
decision-making authority. The defining characteristic
for this model is that decision making is distributed
close to the origin of issue. For example, a requirement
raised for the laboratory system at Hospital A would

be decided by management at Hospital A, not by executives and the CIO at the corporate offices. The corporate CIO only has dotted-line responsibility for the MIS director at each entity. The MIS director of each entity directly reports to an executive within his specific entity (e.g., the MIS director of Hospital A reports to the chief financial officer of member Hospital A).

■ *Virtual IS Model.* Shown in Figure 7.4, this model could be a derivation of any functional IS organization chart. This model can be applied when you have established a close working relationship between your health care enterprise and the outside suppliers of IS solutions and services. Organizations apply this model when they need ready access to resources that are limited within their organization and difficult to obtain on short notice. IS professionals with specific skill sets, an automated rapid-application development methodology, and an installed object-oriented data repository might be examples of tools that could be made available through a virtual IS arrangement. Remember, a virtual IS arrangement allows your IS shop to be deeper in resources on an on-call basis.

■ *Autonomous Operating Units under One Executive Management Team Model.* Shown in Figure 7.5, this organization model is structured as an integrated delivery system. It has well-defined lines of decision making. The executive management team is usually high caliber and has a vision that is often understood in the communities it serves. From a technological perspective the integrated delivery system looks to apply common IS solutions across operating units as a stated business direction. The IS shop(s) in this model often supports both owned and affiliated entities. IS decision making rests with the corporate CIO. The CIO in this model needs to function as a member of executive management and take on similar characteristics to those outlined later in this chapter.

■ *Autonomous Operating Units with Loose Management Affiliation.* Shown in Figure 7.6, this organization model is a derivation of the previous model. This model becomes prevalent when the integrated delivery system has truly autonomous regions or a national presence. This model functions best when there is a collaborative operational environment with end-point decisions residing within the operating unit. IS guidance and oversight is typically facilitated through some form of management council with no formal enforcement methodology. The corporate CIO has few direct reports. Good corporatewide decision making is dependent on the degree of common corporate culture exhibited throughout the organization.

The Models and Factors to Consider

Outsource Model. Consider When (see Figure 7.1)

■ Acquisition of specialized IS talent is too difficult.

■ Management needs dramatic improvements in service levels.

■ The culture of the existing IS department is not responsive to mission-critical initiatives.

■ Management desires to accurately predict IS expenditures over a long period of time.

■ Executive management is hands-off with IS but wants high degree of accountability.

■ Management seeks a means of capital infusion into the organization.

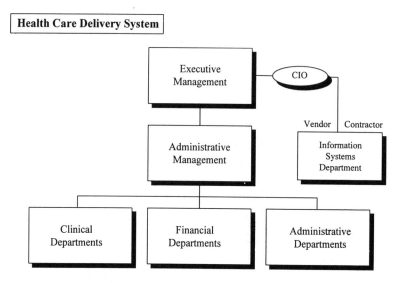

Figure 7.1   *Outsource Model*

Centrally Flat Hierarchy Model. Consider When (see Figure 7.2)

- ■ Allocation of scarce IS resources is critical.
- ■ Information management initiatives tend to drift away from intended objectives during implementation.

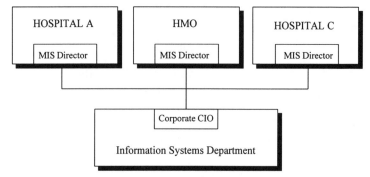

Figure 7.2   *Central Flat Hierarchy Model*

■ Strong leadership is required to adhere to a results orientation.

■ Middle-layer IS management and staff have difficulty reaching consensus.

Centralized Oversight Model. Consider When (see Figure 7.3)

■ Maximizing end-user responsiveness when economies of scale can be gained through parent affiliation.

■ Optimizing knowledge transfer of similar information requirements exists.

■ Required IS knowledge differs significantly among affiliated entities.

■ Centralized decision making cannot be made in a timely fashion.

■ There is no enterprisewide funding capability.

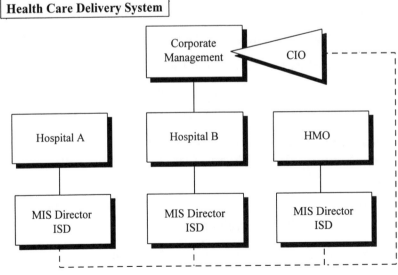

Figure 7.3 *Centralized Oversight Model*

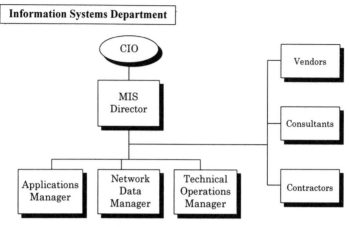

Figure 7.4　*Virtual IS Model*

Virtual IS Model. Consider When (see Figure 7.4)

- ■ Organization has intermittent demands for unique skill sets.

- ■ Desiring risk sharing with IS deployment.

- ■ Strategic alliance exists with your vendor or consultant.

- ■ Overhead costs are high for in-house expertise.

- ■ Pushing the technology envelope for your own organization by implementing cutting-edge IT solutions.

Autonomous Operating Units under One Executive Management Team Model. Consider When (see Figure 7.5)

- ■ Economies of scale can be leveraged to advantage of IS acquisition and rollout.

- ■ Desiring single point of accountability.

- ■ Cross-entity issues and resolution and solution implementation are focal points.

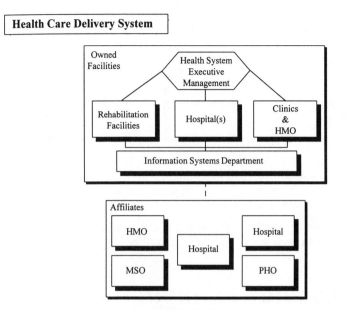

Figure 7.5 *Autonomous Operating Units under One Executive Management Team Model*

■ End-user service delivery is evaluated on personal contact and hands-on execution.

■ Clear lines of communication are necessary to ensure vision execution.

Autonomous Operating Units with Loose Management Affiliation Model. Consider When (see Figure 7.6)

■ Information exchange and issue identification is central objective.

■ Consensus building is natural to the organization and management participants.

■ Common vision can be executed through multiple means.

■ Common IS foundation must be tailored to accommodate end-user assimilation.

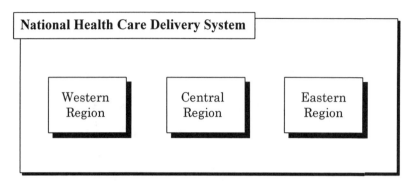

Note: Figure 7.5 would be pictured within each regional box.

Figure 7.6   *Autonomous Operating Units with Loose Management Affiliation Model*

Tools and Techniques

To forge a fully responsive IS organization, the CIO needs to develop new capabilities, new skill sets, and new degrees of precision and discipline within his staff. Building seamless patient or member recognition systems across a myriad of legacy systems just cannot be done without people who understand how to construct enterprisewide views of the mission-critical data sets. Developing robust enterprisewide networks to support the data flows for all of the enterprisewide applications requires the ability to leverage technology for best performance while providing maximum tolerance for network disruptions. Having resources within the IS department that understand the needs of the new clients, (e.g., medical informatics) becomes essential to meeting client expectations.

New skills and capabilities, however, will not be sufficient. As the metrics of performance shift toward the new yardstick, the criteria for competent project management and maintaining effective client relationships will become more stringent. New tools, together with a heightened sense of professional discipline in applying the tools, will become the norm. Every project will have a charter. The concept of delivering a project on time and on budget will take on new relevancy in the IS shop. Every team leader will know how to facilitate interorganizational work sessions. Every team will focus on delivering the benefits of technology to the organization.

In this section we explore ideas for developing the organization's functional capabilities, and project management capabilities.

Functional Capabilities

Technical capabilities, at an early point in HIN evolution, will need to expand beyond those required to support existing legacy systems. The enterprisewide nature of the new requirements will add a dimension of complexity that can only be addressed with more disciplined, structured approaches to networking, data management, integration, and informatics, as described below.

Components

From a functional perspective the IS organization chart will most likely evolve along the lines of Figure 7.7. Within that framework key components necessary to support the entire enterprise will include:

■ *Medical Informatics Consulting Services.* This group will focus on client services. These are the people who understand client environments and needs, who translate the needs into systems requirements, who become client advocates, and who are focused on finding ways to deliver technology benefits. This group will be prospecting in other industries and other environments for enabling tools and emerging technologies. This group will also be responsible for supporting enterprisewide applications.

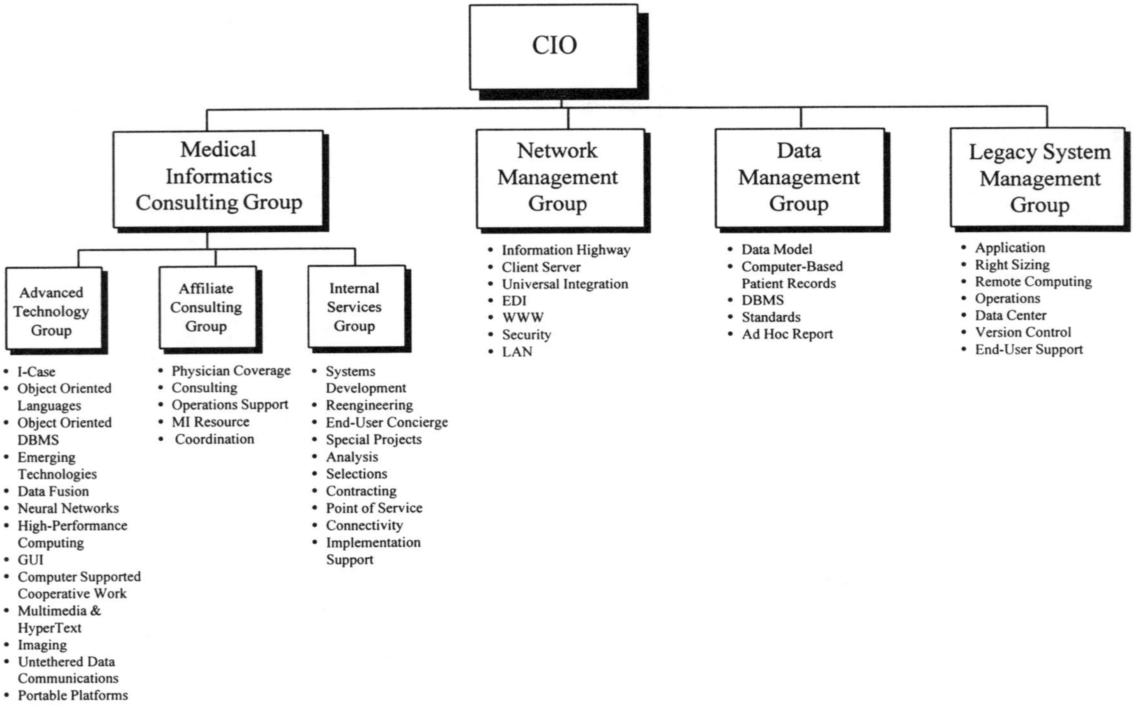

188

Figure 7.7 *Conceptual Functional Organizational Model for Department of Information Systems*

- *Network Management Services.* This group will build, operate, and maintain the enterprise's information highways. Implementing a wide area network (WAN), providing access to the Internet (e.g., World Wide Web), and developing robust local area networks (LANs) will be this group's major activities. This group will also grapple with the state-of-the-art issues in client-server technologies (e.g., replication servers) as they forge fault-tolerant networks that can move data fast enough to meet the clinical user's expectations. This will be the group that implements the universal interface engine (UIE) to link the myriad legacy systems to provide seamless patient or member recognition and enterprisewide scheduling capabilities. This group will be responsible for implementing the enterprisewide security functions.

- *Data Management Services.* This group provides the architectural services necessary to ensure that the enterprise has access to mission-critical data sets. In the planning mode this group builds data models of the enterprise requirements, legacy systems capabilities, seamless systems capabilities, and interfacing requirements to make it all work. In the control mode this group monitors the implementation of interfaces, new releases, data access, and usage. Members become the internal auditors, both in terms of who gains access to what data and in terms of ensuring that the quality of the data itself is consistent with its intended usage. This is the group that will referee the issues regarding how to use data fields consistently across the enterprise (e.g., whom do we define as the attending physician in the enterprisewide view of data?).

- *Legacy Systems Services.* This group is primarily responsible for supporting and operating installed legacy systems in each part of the enterprise and comprises the bulk of today's typical IS organization. These professionals must concentrate on high availability, application reliability, consistent daily production operations, version control, and hardware and operating systems performance tuning. This is the group that provides day-to-day support to the user community for routine services. This group will be challenged to deliver superior services at lower costs. This group will become an early target for consolidation across the enterprise (i.e., the corporate data center).

Process Redesign

Information services as an organization needs to become involved in the enterprise reengineering initiatives as early as possible. While the traditional IS perspective has been to wait for the user to define his requirements, this will not work in the future because:

- The reengineering user does not know what capabilities IS can or cannot provide or what data is actually available or not available in other parts of the enterprise.

- The user expects someone else (i.e., the CIO) to be responsible for getting him the data he needs when he needs it and from wherever it needs to come from, even if it does not exist anywhere today!

- The user may need help translating his operational needs into information system needs/capabilities.

- The user probably does not know how to leverage the technology to deliver maximum benefits to his organization.

- The user may not be able to visualize the situation beyond his own organizational boundaries.

Information services has the unique ability to help these clients look beyond their organizational boundaries (an enterprisewide perspective), inject the realities of the market-place into the dialogue (what's real, what's vaporware), and focus energy on maximizing the benefits of shared data and enterprisewide capabilities. But this will only happen if IS constructs a way to gain early admittance to the reengineering initiatives through the governance processes described earlier.

Short-Term Tactics

What can the CIO do, rather quickly, to begin building these functional capabilities? We suggest an initial focus for each domain.

- Acquire credible client-focused personnel to begin working with enterprisewide clients. Immerse them in the major reinventing and reengineering initiatives. It is very likely these people are already present within the enterprise, but not necessarily within the current IS organization.

- Acquire a network architect to start the WAN/LAN and client-server design processes. At the scale of an enterprisewide network, supporting seamless services at 40, 50, or even 100 sites, the technical issues are an order of magnitude larger than experienced in today's hospital-based environment. There will be little toler-ance for a long learning curve. There will be no toler-ance for an unstable network. It is unlikely that the capability to design competently at this scale resides within the present organization.

- Acquire resources to lead development of the enter-prise data model. The scale of the data modeling effort is likely to exceed the experience of most health care-based IS shops. Not only will there be little tolerance for a long learning curve, but there's also just a lot of work to get done before the enterprise can begin to leverage the data it already owns.

■   Take a close look at the options for delivering highly reliable daily operations at an enterprise level. The real issues to focus on are client-service levels and costs. The service levels are likely to range from great to lousy; the costs will all be too high. This is a key area where consolidation can enhance both service levels and costs.

Focus on Project Orientation

Project management is the discipline typically used to design and deploy new capabilities to the IS client. Projects provide the infrastructure needed to organize the people, coordinate the work effort, facilitate communications, coordinate resource allocations, and resolve issues. As the evolving HIN cranks out project after project, the CIO and his major clients will expect new levels of consistency, reliability, and competence in project management.

What Is New and Different?

Project plans have always been the basic management vehicle for carrying out IS work. So, what's different today?

■   *New Tools and Techniques.* Over the last five years project management software has matured substantially, yet it has only been used for very large projects typically led by vendors or consultants. The learning curve still seems to impede universal use by the IS organization. Creating interorganizational work teams has become an organizational norm in the client setting, thanks to the intense focus on continual quality improvement over the last five years. That, however, does not mean the IS organization universally embraces the approach. New emphasis on the use of project charters—again from the improvement arena—brings new clarity to the mission, objectives, structures, and roles of the players in projects. Getting up-front agreement to the charter is the current focus; creating a dynamic project charter that can adapt to the changing requirements will be the future challenge.

■ *Accountabilities Are Different.* At the scale of HIN initiatives, the organizational stakes are very high; the capital dollars involved are 10 times those of the typical IS project; and the consequences of not meeting objectives or timeliness are obvious to everyone. The stakeholders are totally dependent on the CIO to deliver the services they must have to meet their own objectives. There is no place for the CIO to hide if IS does not get things done right the first time.

Imperatives for the CIO

To echo the last paragraph, the CIO needs *highly reliable* project management processes that will deliver results within the time frames and costs committed by the enterprise. To make that happen, the CIO must instill a new level of discipline in the management of every IS project. Project charters, computer-aided work plan management, and collaborative work processes will have to become the institutional standards. They must be woven into the very fabric of the IS culture as "This is the way we work together. . . ."

Clarity about consequences of not meeting project objectives needs to be part of the project dialogue as well, not as a threat but as a vehicle to clarify the core needs that absolutely must be met to crystallize the sense of urgency. The CIO must lead these dialogues, making them legitimate, relevant conversations and demonstrating his full commitment to the team's success.

Project leaders must have the skills to work effectively in this highly charged environment. At this scale, project leaders can no longer rely on control strategies to be successful. Collaborative techniques developed for large-scale organizational change projects must become the primary vehicles for empowering the large numbers of people involved in these initiatives. Interpersonal skills will be a dominant discriminant between effective and ineffective project leaders.

CIO and Client Perspective

Clients will presume that this level of competency already exists within the IS organization. This is part of their yardstick. Yet, we find the typical health care CIO believes that managing the organizational change process is the client's job, not his. Again, it's the distinction between delivering technology and delivering benefits of technology. We believe that the CIO must be committed to work *in collaboration* with his clients to deliver the benefits of technology. To make that happen, the CIO's resources need to effectively guide the client in every aspect of the initiative.

The People Part

Up to now we have focused on the nature of the environment, the requirements, and the client perspectives. Now we will explore implications for the people who actually do this work.

Critical Skills

To accomplish the HIN agenda, IS resource experts will be needed in such areas as:

- *Data Modeling.* Including enterprisewide sharing of clinical data in the computerized patient record (CPR) and seamless patient or member recognition applications.

■ *Interface Engines.* Including enterprisewide movement of data among the legacy systems and new enterprise solutions and into and out of the enterprisewide clinical data repository.

■ *Network Architecture.* Including design of highly robust, scalable networks capable of supporting mission-critical clinical applications.

■ *Medical Informatics.* Including understanding the clinical decision maker's environment and needs.

■ *Internal Client Consulting.* Including bringing the disciplines of project management, client management, and effective interpersonal skills to the organization.

■ *Reengineering.* Including the disciplines and techniques of reinventing and repositioning both the business and clinical processes across the entire enterprise.

■ *Business Change Implementation Techniques.* Including the techniques for deploying large-scale business and clinical work process changes across the entire enterprise.

Our premise is that asking people to do this kind of work without access to the subject-matter experts is an invitation to frustration and eventual failure. We've also touched on the more universal skill sets that will be needed by every IS professional in this chaotic environment.

■ Ability to lead projects through collaborative group processes.

■ Ability to tolerate significant levels of ambiguity and changing requirements.

■ Ability to facilitate resolution of highly charged interpersonal situations and organizational conflicts.

■   Ability to stay focused on what is important, not what is urgent (see "Effecting the Transition" at the conclusion of this chapter).

■   Ability to learn from every experience.

Along the way we have offered thoughts on how these skills and capabilities will contribute to the success of enterprisewide IS initiatives. We have touched on whether the CIO is likely to find these skills within his department or enterprise. We believe that two interlocking questions confront the CIO:

■   Should I recruit from the marketplace (internal to the enterprise or externally) or develop my existing people?

■   How fast do I have to deliver the capability to my clients?

The answer to the second question dictates the answer to the first. The capabilities need to be timely enough to be able to be deployed when needed, which means an understanding of what is happening at the enterprise (HIN) level is critical. The CIO needs the governance processes to provide early warning. An understanding of the professional goals and objectives of the current IS staff is also necessary.

Reorganization and Retention

By now it should be apparent that the IS organization chart will be changing, probably as often as the enterprise organization chart. Each merger will bring new people, new clients, and new expectations. What will it be like to actually work in this turbulence?

The answer to this question depends on the corporate CIO's leadership skills. To use an analogy, when you board a commercial airliner, you assume a level of technical competence in the pilot and crew. You expect them to get us safely from airport to airport. Along the way, you expect them to be friendly, somewhat flexible, and certainly focused on your comfort and safety. So, what is your reaction when the ride gets rough? If the pilot has conveyed a sense of competence, you are willing to trust him to get you through and find smoother air. If not, you get sweaty palms.

The corporate CIO will need to demonstrate the same sense of competence to his own staff. There will be turbulence. Whether they get sweaty palms or renewed confidence depends on three fundamental factors.

- Do they believe the CIO has the leadership skills to reset the compass when needed?

- Do they believe the CIO has the skills to form a very resilient organizational culture, one that relies on a core set of values to guide its reactions to the turbulence?

- Do they have confidence in themselves, in their skills, and in their relationships?

Our advice to the corporate CIO is this: *Focus your energy and talents on developing a highly resilient organizational culture. This is the single most effective way to encourage your high performers to ride out the turbulence.*

The traditional approaches of high salaries, exotic titles, and inflated roles will not get the job done in what Peter Vail describes as the "permanent white water" of today's environment.[1]

The CIO's Role

A fundamental expectation for a CIO is to lead the IT professionals within an organization. IT professionals want to, and will, perform for a good CIO. Conversely, a poor or weak CIO is the single greatest disrupter to an IT department. Lack of direction, indecisiveness, and poor communications can be the demise of an IT organization. The CIO sets the tone for how the IT department is perceived throughout the enterprise.

Until the integrated delivery networks and the merger-affiliation activities stabilize and mature, the CIO will constantly encounter changing needs and priorities for IT support. The IT department, and specifically the CIO, will be measured by the new yardstick discussed earlier through this transitionary period.

Understanding the Strategic Agenda

The strategic agenda for the health care industry has been set for the next several years. This agenda is represented by the graphics in Chapter 2. The CIO will need to immerse himself in understanding the future state of health care delivery to implement organizational plans necessary to meet the user needs within this agenda. *He must become one of its architects.*

Demonstrations of IT technical competence alone will not be sufficient. The CIO, during the planning process, must bring to the organization an understanding of advanced technologies and how they can be deployed to support the vision. Knowledge of the current state of the applications marketplace, although critical, will not satisfy the sense of urgency for new capabilities and new levels of integration. Academic and practical understanding of such concepts as managed care, outcomes management, physician-practice strategies, as well as other areas discussed throughout this book, will enable the CIO to design and implement an IT organizational infrastructure that can remain responsive to changing demands.

The New Reality

The CIO's IT organization must interact with the sponsors, architects, and advocates of specific IT initiatives. These initiatives will emerge, blossom, fade, and move on as their agendas are tried, evaluated, and either incorporated or cast aside in the continual search for solutions that can address these business and medical imperatives. Although this has always been a part of the health care CIO's environment, the pace at which this occurs will be astonishing. For the CIO in the midst of this, several themes impacting the IT organization are likely to emerge.

While a corporation's strategic goals may tend to remain relatively consistent, the tactics and technologies for achieving those goals will be constantly changing. The myriad of concurrent IT initiatives will appear insurmountable and may result in conflicting project objectives. The IT department must be able to effectively prioritize and accommodate flexible and shifting staffing assignments. The communication of tactical changes moves quickly; therefore, IT should consider adopting a "quasi-continual" improvement approach for internal communications.

Within the IT community there will remain an intense competition for the highly talented people who can also tolerate the ambiguity of the health care environment. Health care corporations for the time being will be constantly reorganizing and redeploying resources. New leaders, therefore, or familiar leaders in unfamiliar roles, will now be driving the agendas for change. Reemphasizing an earlier point, the IT organization must align its structures to support the evolving business enterprise. The CIO, therefore, must be familiar with and have trained resources in the subject matter of process reengineering.

The traditional information systems steering committee structure will have difficulty providing sufficient direction to the CIO, both because its membership is changing constantly and because the change agenda will remain in flux during this transition period of the industry. In the short term executive management should experiment with new ways to communicate with and provide guidance to the IT organization. As discussed earlier, it is paramount to address governance related to any oversight committee during any IT reorganization exercise.

Responsibilities and Characteristics

Simply put, many of today's CIOs may not be up to the challenges facing them. So how does executive management or self-appraisal determine which IT executives are up to tomorrow's challenges? The following points and observations are intended to provide insights into some of the qualities successful CIOs need.

The CIO needs to be a leader, teacher, salesman, and motivator. Without a doubt the biggest transition in skills is from manager to leader. Most of today's CIOs are managers. Long-term leadership traits at this executive level will be more valued than management skills. Leaders need to establish the vision and communicate direction. Managers focus on being action oriented and finding people who can get the task at hand done. Management skills can be supplemented with strategic hires within the IT department, but the organization's ability to adopt and absorb technological change must ultimately come from a CIO's leadership.

A recent article about leadership by David Cooper of Knight-Ridder newspapers pointed out that leadership has numerous ingredients: intellect, determination, patience, commitment, consistency, vision, kindness, boldness, the ability to focus on important broad issues, and above all, the ability to motivate people and persuade them to accept your ideas (as teacher, salesman, motivator). Cooper used these traits to evaluate the leadership abilities of the presidents of the United States.[2] The same traits should be used to evaluate the leadership skills of CIOs.

Does the CIO understand the implications of the pending strategic agenda within the industry? Again, the CIO needs to be one of the architects implementing that agenda for his organization. To be fully accepted as one of the architects, the CIO will need to demonstrate the following:

- Commitment to delivering the benefits of technology, not just installing computer equipment.

- A sense of urgency expressed in the future-state vision.

- Understanding of the HIN future-state vision.

■ Understanding of how the HIN delivers health care services.

■ Understanding of the key enablers and barriers to transforming the current IT organization into its future-state HIN.

■ Ability to bring together people with diverse viewpoints, helping them develop a common vision to guide the deployment of information technology.

■ Openness to the possibility that his own agendas are inconsistent with those of the emerging and evolving organization.

■ Willingness to continually learn.

■ Willingness to make the tough decisions in a timely fashion.

Effecting the Transition[3]

Stephen R. Covey's book, *The Seven Habits of Highly Effective People,* can serve as a methodology to enable CIOs to identify and focus on the tasks necessary to reorganize their IS departments to better implement an enterprise's strategic agenda. For those who have not read the book, Covey states that effective people and organizations need to establish priorities that are related to fulfilling their mission, roles, and goals. Covey has a time-management model divided into four quadrants: Quadrant one items are important and urgent; Quadrant two items are important but not urgent; Quadrant three items are urgent but not important; Quadrant four items are both not important and not urgent.

Items in Quadrant one are situations such as important meetings or matters you must address; otherwise you do not survive within the organization. Quadrant three items are things such as unanswered mail or someone else's priorities that do not further the firm's mission. These items typically cut into the time you have available to dedicate to mission-critical priorities. Quadrant four is reflective of unnecessary or ill-prepared meetings. If you had concentrated on Quadrant four tasks all day, at the end of the day you would have felt like you had been very busy but had not accomplished anything. Covey describes Quadrant two tasks as those things that are "important but not urgent." Quadrant two items usually have significant relevance to an organization's ability to achieve its mission and goals.

Covey believes that effective people and organizations must focus attention on tasks in Quadrant two. IS organizations need to become Quadrant two oriented. Tasks not contained in Quadrant two that are deemed urgent typically require reactionary management intervention to resolve. In essence, these items create the departmental fire fighting we see in many organizations. To effect an organizational realignment will require IS shops to get out of the fire-fighting mode. IS professionals tend to focus on their users' urgent needs. Covey believes the truly important tasks are seldom really urgent matters. He also states that everything cannot be an A item on your priority list. Therefore, the number of truly important tasks and projects should be limited.

For example, if the HIN is central to your enterprise's future mission, three important but not urgent tasks for the IS department to initiate include:

- Aligning your IT organizational model with your business enterprise's organization structure.

- Reengineering your core care-delivery processes as outlined in Chapter 3.

- Implementing the IT infrastructure to support the enterprise, as discussed in Chapter 2.

Now is the time to identify and begin addressing your Quadrant two activities. The CIO who takes these steps is well on the way to being highly effective, producing exceptional results, and being perceived as leading the transition to health care's future state.

Summary

As we have seen, the rapid, almost explosive rate of change occurring in health care delivery mechanisms is going to place unprecedented demands on IS organization and its leadership. As it becomes apparent that information technology is the most important enabler for the integrated delivery system's reengineering initiatives, the pressures will grow even more. The CIO will be expected to collaborate effectively at the highest levels of the enterprise. He will be expected to develop a fully responsive IS organization. He will be expected to build an infrastructure that is technically robust, flexible, and cost-effective. And he will be expected to deliver the benefits of technology to the enterprise.

We believe that the core elements of any IS organizational mission and values should emphasize effective collaboration, responsiveness, technical competence, and benefits delivery. The CIO who focuses his energy on these elements will be well positioned to support the enterprisewide transformation of the health care delivery system.

Notes

1. Peter B. Vaill, *Managing as a Performing Art: New Ideas for a World of Chaotic Change* (San Francisco, Jossey-Bass Publishers, 1991).

2. David B. Cooper, "Whatever Happened to Leaders?" *The Charlotte Observer* (December 7, 1994), p. 19A.

3. Stephen R. Covey, *The Seven Habits of Highly Effective People* (S&S Trade, 1989).

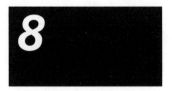

8

Implementation Planning

Overview

Implementation planning consists of identifying all projects necessary to achieve the organization's vision; evaluating these projects in terms of priority, cost, and resource needs; then grouping, budgeting, and scheduling the projects over the next several years. Until an organization inventories all of the technology, application, process, and organizational projects necessary to move from the current state to the future vision, it lacks a complete understanding of the effort's scope and breadth.

Add to this the estimated costs, time frames, and resource needs for each project, and the organization has the information necessary to determine over what period of time the vision is realizable and what it will take in terms of dollars, manpower, and time to achieve. Once costs, skill sets, and time frames are identified, the organization can group projects based on priority, budget, and resource availability.

A sound implementation plan can mean the difference between success and failure in achieving the vision. Not only does the implementation plan act as a tool against which progress towards the vision can be measured, but it is also dynamic, allowing the incorporation of new information, new technologies, and new applications as they become available.

Which Projects First and When?

Before deciding on which projects to schedule and when, the organization needs to identify the projects necessary to accomplish its technology plan and rank their priority, identify the high-level costs and resource needs of each one, and then match the projects against budget and resource plans to determine which projects to implement and when.

Identifying Projects

Implementation planning begins with the identification of projects necessary to achieve the organization's vision. This exercise encompasses mapping the current technology to the future technology plan, identifying the incremental steps between the two, and grouping these steps into executable projects.

As projects are identified, a brief, high-level statement of the scope of each project should be developed. These statements should clearly define what will be included in the project and what will not—the boundaries of the project. These high-level project statements not only help ensure that all projects have been identified (i.e., by better assuring that a project is not thought to encompass more than it does), but also provide the foundation for future detailed project planning.

Projects may be application, technology, process, or organization oriented. Application projects are best identified by listing all potential technology applications in the future organization, whether or not the application exists in today's organization. A list of the applications can best be generated by grouping individual applications into major systems categories such as patient management (e.g., registration, scheduling, medical records, etc.), patient accounting (e.g., billing and managed care systems), financial information (e.g., general ledger, accounts payable, materials management, etc.), personnel information (e.g., time and attendance, payroll, human resources, etc.), desktop applications (e.g., word processing and spreadsheet systems), enterprisewide systems (e.g., optical storage and electronic mail systems), and so on.

Technology projects consist of those projects that bridge the gap between the current architecture and the future technology architecture. In most cases, technology projects support application projects: desktop applications need desktop hardware, printers, and local area networks on which to operate; geographically dispersed points of care need a wide area network for receipt, storage, and transfer of patient information. Both technology examples include the hardware, wiring, communication software, and so on, necessary to finalize the project.

Process projects support retooling information flows throughout the organization. Three particular examples illustrate this point: Today's health care mergers and subsequent back office consolidation and centralization require rethinking the work flows as well as staffing levels to implement the new organizations. System implementation projects automatically establish the need to retool processes to best use new system(s) features and functionality. Managed care and the new competitive marketplace are requiring health care organizations to better understand the components of their costs and reduce or eliminate redundant, duplicative, or inefficient processes in order to remain viable.

People projects are those that transform the current organization into the optimal organizational structure. New applications, technology, and processes may require updated skill sets and new or revised organizational structures. Other influences affecting today's organizations include:

- Organizational streamlining or flattening of the organization.

- System usability, allowing for more user involvement in system operation and maintenance and less reliance on the information systems department.

- Today's changing technology focus, which is calling for database and telecommunication specialists as well as system analysts (not programmers).

See Chapter 7: The People Part for a more detailed discussion of information technology organizations.

Ranking Projects

Once the projects are identified, they must be ranked by priority. This means evaluating each project against predetermined criteria and assigning a score or rank. The criteria used to rank projects may be generated from various sources, including the organization's business strategy, user objectives, system dependencies, and economic principles. These criteria should have been determined early in the planning process.

Based on the projects' evaluations against criteria, they can be grouped into those meeting most of the criteria, those meeting many of the criteria, and those that are limited. These groupings can then be identified as high-, medium-, and low-priority projects, respectively.

High-priority projects are those that are most consistent with the organization's business strategy and that meet most of the overall business requirements. These are the projects that will not only provide the organization with the biggest bang for its buck, but will also, once implemented, move the organization much closer to its ultimate technology vision. Figure 8.1 provides a sample format for ranking projects.

At this juncture three important points must be made. First, it is paramount to get user buy in of the project rankings. Without user buy in, getting the organization to sacrifice short-term rewards in order to make progress towards the longer-term vision will be difficult, if not impossible. Only with user support is the long-term vision realizable.

Second, it may be difficult to agree on project rankings because each potential project is a high priority to someone in the organization. It is essential, no matter how difficult, to rank the projects as objectively as possible. Only then can the organization begin to accomplish those projects that are truly critical to its future.

Last, there is probably no way the organization can implement all high-priority projects at once, due to resource and cost constraints. An organization will find that a mixture of high-, medium-, and sometimes even low-priority projects will be combined into one year's budget and over a several-year planning horizon. This is not bad because all these projects move the organization closer to the vision. It is important, however, to

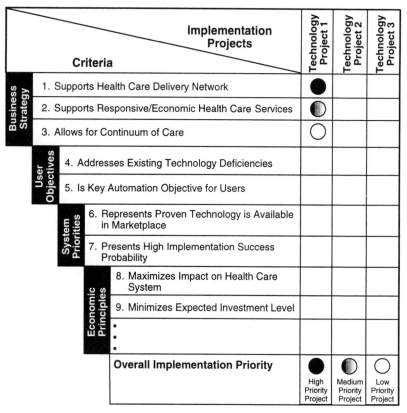

Figure 8.1   *Project-Ranking Schematic*

acknowledge that completing all the high-priority projects immediately is probably unrealistic.

Cost Considerations

Once the projects are identified and ranked, each project must be costed at a high level. The cost breakdown includes onetime project costs as well as ongoing costs. Figure 8.2 on pages 212–213 shows a sample cost breakdown.

Enough detail should be provided in the cost summary to understand each cost item. Further, the cost summary should also include estimates of project time frames and how the costs will be spread over each year of a multiyear project. Uncommitted resource skill sets needed to complete the project, as well as other potential project risks, should be identified with recommendations as to how the organization plans to overcome the particular resource shortage or risk.

As the costs are identified for each project, development of the implementation plan can begin. By matching implementation projects against annual budget estimates, a three- to five-year implementation plan can be constructed.

Other Considerations

Other considerations besides cost affect the scheduling of projects in the final implementation plan. Dependencies, related projects, and the need for short-term wins are three considerations.

Certain projects are dependent on other projects, and these dependencies must be considered in scheduling. For example, patient management, order entry, and results reporting systems are all dependent on an admission/discharge/transfer (ADT) system. Thus, if all of these systems are to be replaced, ADT must be implemented first.

In another situation it may not make sense to execute one project without executing another closely related project. This can be thought of in terms of including an application in the implementation of a vendor suite of applications even though the current application functions as required. For example, if an organization is implementing a single vendor's solution for general ledger, accounts payable, human resources, and payroll applications, it may make sense to implement the vendor's materials management application as well because of its close linkage to the accounts payable application (e.g., vendor database, three-way matching abilities, etc.).

At the start of technology plan implementation, it is important to keep the organization's motivation and good will intact.

INFORMATION SYSTEMS PROJECTED BUDGET WORKSHEET

APPLICATION	PROJECT STATUS/ PRIORITY	IS RANK	RESOURCES (FTEs)	TIME FRAME	ESTIMATED PROJECT FUNDING LOW	HIGH	ESTIMATED FUNDING 1996	1997	1998	1999	2000
Technical & Platform Projects											
Define & Implement Network Strategy	High	3	NM (.75),NA(.75) OA (.5),OM (.1)	Ongoing	$500,000	$800,000	$250,000	$200,000	$150,000	$100,000	$100,000
Rollout/Upgrade end user workstations		9			$100,000	$200,000	$150,000	$100,000			
Interface Engine	High	4									
- Hardware & Software			OM(.1),NA(.1) PG(.1)	3M	$150,000	$200,000	$150,000				
- Selection					$25,000	$30,000	$25,000				
- Implement and Enhance Interfaces (Radiology & Pharmacy)			PG(.5),NA(.1)	4M - 6M	$25,000	$30,000	$25,000				
Electronic Mail	High	3									
- Selection			NM (3)	2M	$50,000	$60,000	$50,000				
- Implementation			HD (.5),OA (.5)	12M							
Office Management (WP,Spread, DB)	High										
- Selection			NM (25)	2M	$15,000	$20,000	$15,000				
- Implementation			HD (.5),CE (.5)	6M							
IS Technical Staff Training					$30,000	$50,000					
System Enhancements and Upgrades											
General Accounting		8									
- General Ledger	High		SA (3)	2M	$50,000	$60,000	$50,000				
- Fixed Assets enhancements	High			4W	$50,000	$60,000	$50,000				
Report Writer/Upload/Download data	High										
- Select			OA(.2),(OM,SA)=1	2M							
- Implement			OA(.2),(OM,SA)=1	2M							
New Application Projects											
Patient Management/Accounting											
Managed Care	High	6									
- Hardware & Software			SA (3)	2M	$50,000	$60,000		$50,000			
- Selection			SA (3)	3M - 4M	$20,000	$25,000		$20,000			
- Implementation					$50,000	$60,000		$50,000			
Appointment Scheduling	High	11									
- Hardware & Software			CA (.5)	3M	$350,000	$450,000			$35,000	$300,000	$150,000
- Selection			CA (1)	9M - 12M	$35,000	$45,000				$80,000	$20,000
- Implementation					$80,000	$100,000					
Resource Scheduling (Select w/Appt Sch)											
Enterprise MPI (Select w/Appt Sch)		11									
Patient Care Applications											
Computerized Patient Record											
- Hardware & Software	High	5	CA (.5)	4M	$500,000	$800,000	$60,000	$300,000	$250,000		
- Selection					$60,000	$75,000					
- Order Entry/Results Reporting	High		CA(1),PG(.1)	12M - 18M	$100,000	$130,000		$100,000			
- Implementation											
- Clinical Documentation/Crit Care Paths	Med		CA(1)	12M - 18M	$50,000	$80,000			$50,000		
- Electronic Medical Record/Clinical Rep											
- Clinician Workstations											

Administrative Computing	Priority	Count	Staff	Duration							
Time & Attendance	High	13									
- Selection			SA (1)	3M						$60,000	
- Implementation			SA (1)	2M						$80,000	
Payroll	Low									$10,000	$10,000
Facility Management	Med										
Preventative Maintenance	Med									$15,000	$15,000
Food & Nutritional Support	Low										
Electronic Teleconferencing	Low				$60,000				$60,000		
Consulting Fees									$75,000		
Capitalized Totals					**$270,000**	**$480,000**	**$485,000**	**$820,000**	**$810,000**	**$3,445,000**	**$2,370,000**
IS Salaries											
New Positions											
- Network Analyst					$30,000	$30,000	$30,000	$30,000	$30,000	$35,000	$25,000
- Clinical Analyst (2-3)					$35,000	$35,000	$35,000	$35,000	$35,000	$40,000	$30,000
- Clinical Engineer					$22,500	$22,500	$22,500	$22,500	$22,500	$25,000	$20,000
- Office Automation Analyst					$22,500	$22,500	$22,500	$22,500	$22,500	$25,000	$20,000
Current Positions					$390,000	$390,000	$390,000	$390,000	$390,000	$400,000	$383,000
Maintenance of Current Systems											
Radiology Support				Ongoing							
Pharmacy Support				Ongoing							
Maintenance of Future Systems											
Interface Engine											
Cost Accounting											
Order Entry / Results Reporting											
Office Management Systems											
Appointment Scheduling											
Network Maintenance											
Operating Totals					**$500,000**	**$500,000**	**$500,000**	**$500,000**	**$500,000**	**$525,000**	**$478,000**
Grand Totals					**$770,000**	**$980,000**	**$985,000**	**$1,320,000**	**$1,310,000**	**$3,970,000**	**$2,848,000**

SA - Systems Analyst ; NM - Network Mgr. ; NA - Network Analyst ; LO - Lead Operator;PG - Programmer
OM - Operations Mgr ; HD - Help Desk Tech ; OA - Office Automation Analyst ; CS - Clinical Engineer Supervisor ; PM - PBX Maintenance

Figure 8.2   Cost Breakdown by Project

Scheduling projects that can be quickly completed or have high organizational impact or visibility (or both) will go a long way toward solidifying user buy in of the entire technology plan.

Alternative Migration Strategies

What migration approaches should be used to evolve the integrated delivery system envisioned by the organization? What are the risks? How should an organization select one approach over another?

Three alternative migration strategies, shown in Figure 8.3, are described below. Each of these strategies has a common endpoint—implementation of computer-based patient records, advanced clinical systems, and deliverywide applications—but the steps to get there differ. When selecting an information technology migration strategy able to support the future environment, the following criteria, at a minimum, should be taken into consideration: key management goals, information technology initiatives, the organization's risk tolerance, and market forces (e.g., the anticipated impact of community networks and national health care reform).

Structured Replacement

One migration strategy is structured replacement. The structured replacement migration strategy consists of replacing most of the current systems, including custom-developed applications, and selecting new applications prior to the design and implementation of more sophisticated deliverywide information systems and technologies. The high-level phases of this strategy are:

1. Replacing custom-developed legacy systems and implementing critical strategic systems.

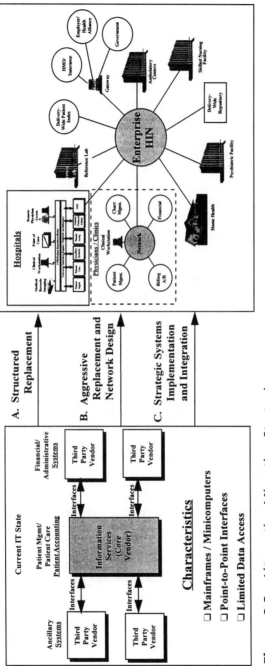

Figure 8.3 *Alternative Migration Strategies*

215

2. Selecting and implementing new systems.

3. Implementing an enhanced network and integration engine.

4. Designing and implementing a computer-based patient record (CPR), advanced clinical systems, and delivery-wide applications.

This strategy allows for a structured building block approach to systems implementation and assumes that replacement systems (legacy and new) exist today and are proven in the marketplace. Moreover, waiting to implement advanced systems and technologies (e.g., advanced clinical systems and CPR) will allow products more time to mature.

This strategy, however, requires a high initial investment in hardware, software, and implementation and delays the integration and implementation of deliverywide solutions. In addition, many of the vendor packages that would replace the core applications (e.g., patient accounting) are still in transition. The risk to the organization undertaking this migration alternative is medium.

Aggressive Replacement and Network Design

A second strategy, aggressive replacement and network design, involves replacing the existing custom-developed systems, selecting and implementing new applications, implementing an enhanced network and integration engine, and implementing the deliverywide solutions as concurrently as possible. The high level phases of this strategy are:

1. Replacing the custom-developed legacy systems, implementing critical strategic systems, and selecting and implementing new systems.

2. Implementing an enhanced network and integration engine and designing and implementing a computer-based patient record, advanced clinical systems, and deliverywide applications.

The major advantage of this strategy over the structured replacement approach is that the implementation of advanced and deliverywide solutions is accelerated. Drawbacks include the extremely high front-end investment in hardware, software, and implementation; the fact that some applications may not be mature enough for implementation; and the extremely high impact on users and the information services department based on aggressive schedules and activities. Overall, this migration alternative is high risk.

Strategic Systems Implementation and Integration

The third migration strategy, strategic systems implementation and integration, involves replacing or acquiring the most critical business support systems prior to the development of a more advanced technical applications environment. Custom-developed legacy systems would not be replaced until later in the migration plan. The high-level phases included in this strategy are:

1. Selecting and implementing new strategic and business support systems (e.g., managed care, practice management, etc.).

2. Implementing an enhanced network and integration engine.

3. Designing and implementing a computer-based patient record, advanced clinical systems, and deliverywide applications.

4. Replacing custom-developed legacy systems.

The advantages of this strategy are that the most immediate system needs are addressed and, therefore, the organization has a greater chance of supporting the business needs on time. Investment costs for core system replacement are delayed with the focus of addressing the critical information needs earlier.

This strategy is less risky than the aggressive replacement approach, yet more risky than the structured replacement approach. Drawbacks include the possibility that mature applications may not be available, or the organization may be an early adopter of some applications. This strategy also requires the organization to continue to use and maintain legacy systems for a longer period of time and to develop temporary interfaces to the integration engine.

Accelerated Implementation

One of today's key challenges for the information systems department is to implement technology faster, better, and cheaper than in the past. Unfortunately, many organizations have not recognized that such increases in speed require investments in such things as infrastructure, team skills in both technical and interpersonal issues, and user investment of time and ownership. However, several accelerators have been identified as key principles that apply to all projects. The degree to which these accelerators are applied, as well as organizational culture, commitment level, and problem type, will determine the amount of acceleration that can be achieved.

Principles

Information technology principles accelerate implementation projects by streamlining project decision making. Information technology principles are basic philosophies regarding how technology should be applied toward achieving business goals. These principles are simple statements of the organization's belief about how it wants to use information technology over the long term. Principles are derived from business goals and corporate strategies and represent the highest level of guidance for technology decision making. Information technology principles are often grouped into user, vendor, and management principles. See Chapter 5—Emerging Standards for examples of each type of principle.

Standards

A standard is an enforced use of a particular set of technologies entitywide. As do principles, standards accelerate the implementation by streamlining decision making. In fact, standards oftentimes "operationalize" the organization's information technology principles. And as discussed in Chapter 5, standards are objective and market driven.

Technology standards are especially critical in obtaining economies of scale such as reducing redundancy between systems and redundancy between job functions throughout the organization.. Today's technology standards include selection of enterprisewide applications (e.g., desktop suite, database, and E-mail packages, etc.), communication protocols (e.g., integration engine, network, etc.), operating systems (e.g., UNIX), and so on. See Chapter 5 for a more detailed look at standards in health care.

User Involvement

In the past a team of computer experts, usually representing the organization's information services department, took responsibility for the analysis, design, and implementation of a system. Users were often invited to participate and served as data gatherers, local knowledge bases, and token representatives in the democratic process of decision making. However, many application projects failed. One reason was that users were not given proper roles on the projects.

Today it's well understood that users should be the focal point of information technology systems development—the project should be user driven. Figure 8.4 represents the different levels in the enterprise that an information technology system must support.

Failing to involve users can lead to part or all of the system not being used, including the following dangers:

■ Too many false assumptions can be made by system developers about the nature of the tasks the system is to

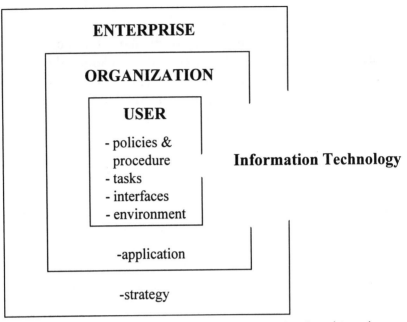

Figure 8.4   *Information Technology—Organizational Levels Supported*

support (even routine tasks can prove more complex than expected).

■ Changes may be resisted because they are felt to be dictated from the outside.

■ Users may be fearful of not being able to cope with the new system.

■ The system developed can be too rigid to cope with local or minor variations and may not meet the need for continuous or additional change over time.

■ Organizational changes may not be planned adequately (e.g., job changes, authority structures, and pay and grading structures).

Involving users leads to greater system acceptance and use. User involvement:

- Ensures that the expertise of the users contributes to analysis of local needs and users' tasks.

- Contributes to good design by identifying current problems, suggesting future trends, increasing the relevance of the system to the tasks performed, increasing the flexibility of the system, and avoiding omissions.

- Reduces fear of the unknown technology and promotes a sense of ownership of the system. This in turn has a very positive effect on levels of user acceptability.

The fact is that user involvement is critical to the success of a process change.

Joint Design Sessions

A joint design session describes an accelerated approach for producing any project deliverable that requires participation of multiple individuals. Joint design sessions are structured workshops that rely on the use of facilitation, visual aids, and documentation tools. In these sessions data is gathered, models are prepared, and feedback is received.

High Performance Teams

High performance teams accelerate implementation. Research on work group and team effectiveness has shown that high performance does not result only from empowering group or team members. In fact, there are a variety of factors involved, all of which must be addressed by the approach the teams use if they are to be successful.

Important questions include:

- How big can and should the teams be?

- What roles should be included in a team or group?

- How are these roles distinguished in order for team members to work cooperatively to achieve mutually agreed targets?

- How do team managers create an environment in which their teams can perform?

The ability to address all aspects of performance is crucial to achieving an accelerated implementation.

Partitioning the Project

Partitioning consists of dividing a large problem or project into smaller, more manageable pieces according to some technical or strategic criteria. It assists in accelerating the process by delivering key functionality early, when it may then be used as a model of the entire completed system. While there may be some management overhead in coordinating multiple partitions, particularly if those partitions are dealt with in parallel, the reduction in complexity offered by the approach, and its promise of early delivery of function, more than offsets such overhead.

Conference Room Pilot

Conference room piloting is an accelerated design approach for implementing software packages. It:

- Configures the base package, using the package parameters and tables.

- Identifies and designs the necessary extensions, bolt-ons, interfaces, and modifications.

- Determines the business transactions that match the package.

- Determines the execution of business transactions by job functions.

The conference room pilot technique attempts to integrate the package as fully as possible into the enterprise, using only the base package features and functions.

Phased Rollout

Implementing in phases has been found to be more effective than a single implementation of the perfect solution for several reasons:

- Technology implementation requires organizational change, and organizational change does not happen overnight. People must have time to acquire new frames of reference and new patterns of behavior.

- Business results are realized as soon as possible. Short- and medium-term solutions do not have to wait for longer-term solutions.

- Each implementation phase can be structured and managed as a separate project.

- Phases of implementation combine short-term attainable levels of ambition with a longer-term vision, and thus radical improvement becomes manageable.

Each subsequent phase builds upon the achievements of the previous one, then targets a higher ambition level. For example, it implements the solution across multiple locations, regions, or countries; implements a more advanced solution; further increases the performance of the targeted business processes; and delivers more business value.

Examples of implementation phases include:

Short-Term Improvements. Identified early on in the project and implemented immediately. Examples include simplifying forms and procedures and eliminating duplicate processes.

Production Pilot. Involves implementing a production pilot in one location. This is a live implementation, complete with hardware installation and data conversion. The environment is controlled, and sufficient resources are available to monitor the implementation and resolve any issues. Typically, user procedures, implementation procedures, package customizations, interfaces, and job designs are refined, based on the experiences of the production pilot, before implementing the system(s) elsewhere.

Rollout. Results in finalizing the cutover to the new systems. The rollout can be accomplished using many different methods, including by location or geographic area, by package module, or by organizational unit.

Balancing Today's Issues with Tomorrow's Goals

How does an organization go about executing its technology plan while maintaining current operations? In other words, how does the organization balance user needs, external requirement changes, and everyday maintenance issues with the priorities of the projects identified in its information technology plan?

Keeping Users Happy

User requests range from minor enhancements to totally new functionality. The costs range from direct cash outlays for equipment to resource consumption such as programmers and technical support. In many cases, user requests can keep the entire information services department busy full time. So how does an organization balance executing projects resulting from user requests (keeping users happy) with those necessary to achieve the organization's longer-term vision?

First of all, without user buy in with the plan, users will not work with the organization to reach the vision. With user support and commitment to the enterprise's technology plan, the information systems organization and users can work together to identify those operational requests that are absolutely necessary, those that can be put on a back burner until budget and resources become available, and those that will just have to wait.

Because users are the technology department's customers, it is important to consider their wish-list projects along with those projects that will advance the enterprise's technology plan. With an eye toward accomplishing the technology plan, user requests to enhance current operations should be kept to a minimum. Only those with definite and immediate financial payback should even be considered. However, if users understand and support the technology plan, they will be more likely to carefully scrutinize their requests and, in turn, to rank highly those projects that support the plan over the majority of their requests.

Meeting Externally Levied Requirements

Projects to support changes in regulatory requirements often take precedence over those projects defined in the technology plan. However, if the technology affected by the regulatory change is supported by the vendor, the vendor will usually provide the update and will require little or no additional organizational resources. If the technology affected by the regulatory change is not supported by a vendor, it is up to the information systems organization to support the requirement, and thus this project will take priority over other technology-plan projects.

Keeping the Current Technology Running

Other types of projects affecting current operations include those that provide for regular maintenance, modernization, and revisions for errors in the technology. Regular maintenance consists primarily of version upgrades that provide additional functionality and possibly corrections to errors found in the previous version of the technology. These upgrades are time consuming to implement and test. Decisions on whether to continue upgrades of the current technology in light of the technology-plan projects must be made and the resulting projects scheduled. If the technology plan calls for replacement of the current technology in the near future, plans for upgrades should be carefully scrutinized and probably halted; if replacement will not occur for some time, then decisions about whether to implement upgrades or to remain on the current version will have to be made and the related projects planned and scheduled if necessary. Again, if the upgrade will be primarily handled by the vendor, whether the technology will be replaced soon is a moot point.

Another aspect of keeping the current technology running is fixing operational errors. Certain resource allotments will have to be made to operate the technology and keep it running. Bug problems not covered by upgrades have to be fixed. Again, a determination must be made between fixes and enhancements. In this case, fixes are the most important because the focus is keeping the current technology operational. Enhancements must be reviewed in light of the technology plan; those to be replaced by new technology should be considered carefully and probably not scheduled; those with a real cost impact should be evaluated as potential projects.

Modernizing current operations is another type of project that needs to be weighed carefully against projects to implement the organization's technology plan. For example, say the organization is implementing an interface engine, and it is determined that spending resource time up front to move certain applications to the interface engine will free up resources in the long run. Then this project, even if it isn't specifically detailed in the technology plan, may be of benefit to the organization without having any direct impact on the plan. Projects like upgrading networks, desktops, printers, and so on, may utilize technology resources but may have a direct payback in terms of increased productivity by those areas receiving the modernization. In most cases, these types of projects will be encompassed in the organization's technology plan. But where they aren't, costs and benefits must be considered in order to determine whether the current operational project should take precedence over the projects identified in the technology plan.

Ingredients of a Successful Project

Many organizations find it difficult to structure, plan, and budget for information technology projects and then meet these estimates with a successfully executed effort—the definition of a successful effort being one that results in a solution that fully meets organizational and user requirements on time and within budget. Many factors can contribute to the success or failure of an information technology project. But the success of any project depends on a few fundamental factors that must be present, as illustrated in Figure 8.5: clear definition, sponsorship, leadership, the project team, organizational adaptability, and planning and control.

Clear Definition

A clear understanding of each project, including expectations, risks, and implementation methodology, is a crucial first step toward executing the enterprise's information technology plan. In defining and understanding project expectations, it is important to identify what will be accomplished and what will not. Completion criteria, budgets, and time frames should all be clearly outlined at a high level. Understanding project expectations, its scope, and its boundaries provides the foundation upon which the project can be planned and executed successfully.

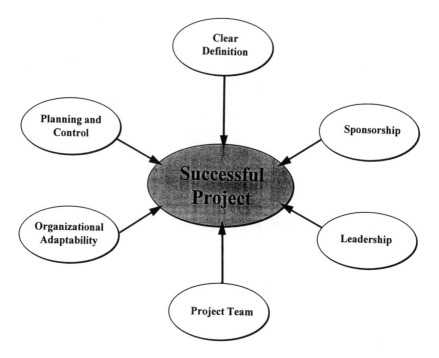

Figure 8.5   *Ingredients of a Successful Project*

When planning for an implementation project, you should identify potential risks, assess their criticality, and develop strategies and programs to manage the risks. Examples of risks in information technology projects are the probability that the project will not finish on time or within budget or, upon completion, that the system will not function as expected. Risks differ from project to project, either in type or criticality, and each project must be looked at individually. Risk assessment should not only take place early in the project but also throughout in order to identify new or previously unidentified risks or to eliminate risks that have been successfully mitigated.

The implementation methodology used to execute technology projects must be clearly defined and understood by at least a subset of project team members. A robust and proven methodology will reduce implementation risk by providing a step-by-step format for project execution. Add to this experienced team members who have successfully used the methodology on other implementation efforts, and you have a recipe for success.

Sponsorship

Sponsorship plays an important role in project success. Source of funding, resource commitment, and organizational backing for a project all are dependent on sponsors. Different levels of sponsorship are critical to the success of an implementation project.

Project Sponsors have the ultimate authority and responsibility for the project. These sponsors are senior executives who have a vested interest in project results, who fund the project, resolve conflicts over policy or objectives, and provide high-level direction. Specifically, at the outset the project sponsors establish reasonable and specific goals, provide the necessary resources, show support for the project, take action on requests, and facilitate the project team's relations with support departments. Project sponsors are also responsible for approving changes during the implementation process, providing additional funding required to absorb the changes, and accepting the new technology at the end of the project. The project sponsors do not need to have implementation experience or detailed knowledge of information technology, since their role is primarily that of a business decision maker for the projects.

Executive Managers are executives within the organization who have a direct responsibility or stake in project results. All user organizations and the information systems department are represented by executive management. Executive management is not only responsible for approving the project team's work throughout the entire project but also for ensuring that the technology that results from the project meets the requirements of and is properly integrated into the organization. Other responsibilities include inspecting project deliverables and making the decision regarding final acceptance of the system.

Resource Coordinators hold management-level roles in the organization and are in some way, shape, or form affected by the project. Resource coordinators support the project primarily by providing staffing for project tasks and subject-matter expertise for the organizational functions for which they are responsible. Resource coordinators serve project sponsors by enhancing organizational commitment.

Leadership

A successful project must have an effective leader. The role of an effective project leader, oftentimes called a project director, includes:

- Reviewing and approving deliverables

- Managing expectations and relationships

- Providing recommendations and not just alternatives

- Involving team members in the decision-making process

- Minimizing outside pressure on the project team

- Providing for team members' personal goals during the project

The project director is not only a leader but also a process manager. As a leader, she is responsible for managing and communicating a clear vision of the project objectives and motivating the project team to achieve them. As a process manager, he must ensure that the right timing, resources, and sequencing of work efforts are applied to create the project deliverables within a given time frame and budget.

Characteristics of an effective leader include experience, flexibility, and sound interpersonal skills. Project sponsors, as well as project team members, will be more apt to follow direction from an experienced leader; simply put, an experienced project director is more credible. Projects, even with carefully and completely documented scopes, are rarely static. Discovery of additional tasks not originally documented in the scope, identification of required functionality thought not necessary at the start of the project, and the loss of seasoned project team members or the addition of new team members all require the project director to incorporate these new tasks and resources into the project plan. Finally, the project director must be able to lead and motivate the project team, manage the project sponsorship relationship, and create a highly productive and synergistic project environment.

The Project Team

The project team is made up of individuals with various skill sets that, in combination, provide the overall skills necessary to successfully implement the project. Users, system analysts, designers, technologists, documentation specialists, and trainers should be on an information technology project team. Members may represent all areas of the organization affected by the implementation effort, including user and technical groups. Although a core project team will support the implementation effort from start to finish, other project team members may be inserted as specialized talent is needed.

Again, technology projects should be user driven. Even if all key users cannot participate in the project directly as project team members, they are important to involve in the implementation project for two reasons. User involvement is essential to ensure that the new technology is designed and integrated in a manner to satisfy user requirements and that the transition to the new technology is straightforward (because the users have been involved and have a stake in the effort). Key users can supplement the project team on an as-needed basis to assist, for example, with the design or decision making regarding functionality. At the very least, all key users should be kept informed throughout the implementation effort about project status and key decisions.

Technology vendors are primarily responsible for the delivery and implementation of purchased technology. In addition, the vendor may support the project team by participating in validation and testing, providing user and technical training, and assisting in conversion activities. Vendors are frequently responsible for the changes to their technology that allow it to be better integrated into the enterprise. The exact nature of the vendor's role and responsibilities on a project should be clearly defined in a contract.

Organizational Adaptability

New technology often causes change in organization structure and culture. Before commencing an implementation project, the enterprise must try to determine the attitudes and responses of people who will actually use the new technology. If senior executives suspect these attitudes are negative, a change management program must be incorporated into and implemented along with the information technology project.

Several strategies can be deployed to assist in the change process: sensitivity to the organization and the cultural changes required by the new technology, identification of the factors that will most likely facilitate or hinder the project, and planning ahead to overcome resistance and anxiety. Some may be unwilling to change, others will be unable to change. Different remedies apply.

Planning and Control

Another aspect of a successful implementation effort is to ensure that the right work gets done the right way, the first time. Planning and controlling the project is one way to accomplish this. The planning process begins by identifying and confirming the business problem to be solved. How to overcome the problem becomes the initial definition of the project. The project scope is then defined, deliverables are identified, and high-level estimates of time frames, required effort, and cost are developed.

Controlling the project is an ongoing process that includes measuring actual progress against the plan and identifying those areas requiring corrective action or adjustments. Project control also encompasses risk management, change management, and quality management. Specifically, developing realistic costs, schedules, and goals; identifying early on potential problems and contingencies to mitigate these problems; controlling change; and communicating—all enable better planning and control of an information technology project.

Summary

Implementation planning is a logical step in reaching any technology goal. As with any type of planning, the more appropriate time is spent deciding and justifying the projects to be accomplished over the next several years, the greater the likelihood of their success. Critical as well is the organization's support of the plan, not only because user support greatly increases any project's potential for success, but also, and more important, sacrifices will have to be made in order to reach the goal. Executing a carefully thought out plan will help an organization move closer to its future vision.

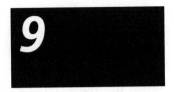

9

Tying It Together

The United States health care industry, as it approaches the twenty-first century, is far different from the one that existed 30 or 40 years ago. In 1960 the health care industry was a mom-and-pop industry comprised of 6,000 or so voluntary, not-for-profit hospitals that served the needs of their communities and 250,000 or so individual physicians, mostly generalists, who served the needs of their neighborhoods and viewed the hospital as a necessary tool in their ability to heal the sick.

The relationship between physician and hospital was one of mutual support and interdependence. Neither could exist without the other, and for the most part it was physicians who sparked, goaded, encouraged, and pushed for changes and improvements to their hospital workshops. Hospital administrators were frequently former clergy or other socially caring managers, sometimes serving part time and at very modest salaries. Few had any professional training in hospital administration.

Many communities were two- or three-hospital towns reflecting the culture of the community and the interests of the physicians. Catholic, Protestant, or Jewish hospitals split the burden of care in many communities, while osteopaths and other medical outcasts were forced to build their own hospitals.

Most patients and their families had to pay for their own care or rely on community largess. Some had access to health insurance partially funded by employers and made available by life insurance companies or cooperative efforts such as Blue Cross plans. Those unfortunate enough to be unable to pay for care were channeled to publicly funded city or county hospitals or to medical schools, where they were used to help train students.

Bad debts were a problem for all hospitals, as was access to capital. The prices charged for services were low, reflecting the hand-to-mouth nature of managing the annual budget. Total spending for health care in the country in 1960 was less than 5 percent of gross national product (GNP). Infant mortality rates were rather high, and the biggest killers were heart attacks, strokes, and cancer. Heart-lung machines, disease-specific antibiotics, disposable plastics, automated blood-testing equipment, continuous monitoring devices, and sophisticated incubators were beginning to come onstream, representing the vanguard of technology that would transform the practice of medicine.

This was the foundation of the modern health care system, and from those relatively simple times, in just 30 short years, the industry has been transformed into the aging juggernaut we have today. During this time America has built a tremendous infrastructure of brick and mortar, technology, and specialized technicians. The country has doubled the annual output of physicians; created a professional hospital management cadre; provided almost universal access to care through Medicare, Medicaid, and generous employer-paid health benefits; and nearly trebled spending as a percentage of GNP. American medicine has conquered or controlled many of the diseases that cut lives short or reduced their quality. But the system is no longer affordable and needs to be restructured to focus more on staying healthy and preventing illness.

Along the way, hospital administrators and the corporate structures within which they operate have become increasingly distanced from patients and their care. In today's modern health care organization, many executives' offices are physically removed from care settings, and a chief executive can literally go for months without visiting a patient in his room. With the government footing the bill for much of the care rendered, health care leaders and practitioners alike have become increasingly preoccupied with how to maximize revenues and how to increase market share.

But the pendulum has begun to lose momentum. Technology, consumer awareness, buyer leverage, and alternative care-delivery models have made obsolete much of the hospital capacity in the country. The health care industry is undergoing a massive restructuring and consolidation, concerned as much with survival and with the bottom line as with the quality of care rendered.

How do all these changes affect the way in which computer technology is used in health care? The computer age has over-lapped the modern hospital age of the last 30 years. Computers began to be used commercially in the 1950s and really became commonplace in hospitals in the 1960s, coincident with the growth spurt fueled by Medicare. Hospital administrators em-braced computers to handle the financial side of health care, and each passing decade has brought a new generation of com-puter technology to help count the numbers. But very little use has been made of computers to directly affect patient care, per-haps reflecting administrators' preoccupation with finances and corporate growth.

To be fair, the same systems that so effectively deal with calculating case-mix adjusted profitability by this or that pa-rameter are pretty much of a hassle to use at the bedside. It's no wonder that so few physicians directly use computers to support the patient-care process. Until very recently computers have been slow and not intuitive. They are *extremely* difficult to use compared to the familiar patient's chart, despite the paper record's shortcomings. No physician has the time to accommo-date the clumsy combinations of passwords, screen flips, and narrow slices of data available on most patient-care systems today. It's so much easier and more flexible to use a pencil and paper. And even if the computer terminal could be made easier to use, the patient-care data available in today's hospital infor-mation systems is incomplete at best.

Does this mean that computers will remain relegated to the back office and to business use rather than clinical use? So long as they remain burdensome to use, the answer will con-tinue to be a resounding yes. But the wrenching change that the industry is undergoing also holds the promise that it will be forced to radically rethink the way computer technology is used. The technology must be made relevant and supportive of the ways health care practitioners do their jobs. Here's why: The blurring of lines between payers and providers, the ratio-nalization of capacity through mergers and affiliations, the transformation of caregivers into multiskilled workers, and a focus on streamlining care to achieve more cost-effective outcomes are all conspiring to redefine the information needs of health care organizations.

Just as the acute-care hospital is becoming obsolete as the epicenter of the health care system, so has the computer technology that supported it. At a time when managers and practitioners need efficient ways to plan, execute, and document care, and to provide caregivers with the information needed to effectively manage a patient over the course of an episode or a lifetime, they are saddled with information systems whose main strength is the ability to account for financial activity after the fact. And the systems used by Provider A do not converse with the systems used by Providers B, C, or D. Just as the health care industry is being transformed, the information systems architecture and infrastructure need to be transformed to support it.

This will take a major investment on the part of health care organizations. Health care executives have been painfully aware of their information systems departments' deficiencies for years, and the pain level has been increasing. Information systems executives in health care have been mostly underfunded and told to make do. Capital budgets have favored clinical technologies, brick and mortar, and service-line development at the expense of information technology. Both CEOs *and* CIOs realize that it can no longer be business as usual when it comes to information technology.

Information systems budgets need to be increased from 2 to 3 percent of operating budgets to 5 to 6 percent over the next couple of years. Skill sets within the information systems department need to be upgraded with the objective of providing better support for users and a more stable, secure, and interconnected network of systems. But there are no assurances, despite the changing requirements for information systems and the increased levels of spending to implement them, that they will be effectively deployed to support the needs of newly formed integrated delivery systems. Senior management can no longer ignore the need to understand or provide leadership and sponsorship to the information systems department. Chief executive, operating, and medical officers must become actively engaged with the chief information officer in guiding the speed and direction of the information systems department. If they don't, the much-needed transformation of information technology will fall short.

It will take most organizations three to five years to reshape their information systems department so that it adds value to the enterprise. Information technology can enable significant improvements in the way patient care is managed. It can reduce errors, increase productivity, shorten lengths of stay, support continuity of care across sites of care and among groups of caregivers, and give new insight into the overall performance of the health care organization. There are numerous examples of each of these among leading organizations, but they do not represent the norm.

Properly deployed information systems can give organizations the ability to manage accounts receivable without reams of paper and from any location. They can allow home care nurses to see more patients and sicker patients in less time than before and without compromising care. They can make it possible, intuitive, and easy for physicians to enter their own orders for tests and therapies within the context of the total picture of what's happening with a patient. They can afford nurses the opportunity to develop tailored plans of care and to easily document activities by noting only the exceptions to the plan. They can eliminate calculation errors for input and output in the critical care unit and reduce overtime. They can help predict the impact of changes in payer mix on the bottom line. They can make it possible for employees to check the status of their benefits and update or change the mix themselves without waiting for someone from human resources to get back to their supervisor. They can make it easier for a patient to gain access to services by precapturing information and sharing it among various departments.

Patients will no longer wonder why they are required to give the same information to several people just to get a simple test done, and they will no longer have to wait what seems an eternity to be served. These same kinds of technology-enabled, streamlined processes have become commonplace in other industries. The next generation of workers and caregivers will be very computer literate and will expect technology support for their day-to-day activities. The same intuitive, interactive, multimedia workstations used by large corporations are beginning to find their way into health care.

But what will it take to make this the norm in health care? As we've shown, there is a structured way to approach the transformation of health care information systems. It first involves developing a clear vision of how the organization will function and what the scope of its activities will be, that is, what direction it will take to become more relevant to its customers. This visioning and direction setting will be the driving force behind information systems planning. One of the most important roles of the CIO in this planning process is to bring to the organization an understanding of advanced technologies and how they can be deployed to support the vision.

The CIO must understand the organization's needs as expressed by the vision and translate these needs into sets of requirements for system design and implementation. Many important technology tools are here today to support the requirements of integrated delivery systems. They include tools such as interface engines for interconnection of systems, and tools to manage data security. The need to flexibly store and access large amounts of clinical and financial data can be met by several commercially available data base products. There are standards that make it easy for users to define their own report and inquiry formats without involving programmers.

PCs as desktop or bedside devices are much more intuitive and easy to navigate than the dumb terminals they replace. Point-and-click access to information, pen-based and voice-actuated entry of data, and real-time reminders and prompts make it possible to expect that physicians will find it easier and more thorough to use the computer than to rely on pencil and paper. In fact, physicians are already seeing these easy-to-use computer techniques employed in the systems they buy to support their individual practices. It's commonplace for their receptionists to be able to keep on top of appointments and billing, and even to electronically submit claims to patients' insurance plans. They have the ability to collect more and more relevant clinical information, and they can easily gain access to various medical libraries, journals, and drug studies to help stay current. Patient instructions are also routinely generated by many of the office practice systems. And I'm sure we've all heard the anecdote about the physician's 12-year-old daughter who was able to generate a summary of patient activity for her mom on a Macintosh on a Sunday afternoon at the office.

Contrast this with what the physician finds at the hospital. At home or at the office he or she can surf the net and send E-mail to a colleague in Scotland. But at the hospital the doctor must rely on a ward clerk to get lab results as long as the system wasn't down last night and they're not still trying to recover—"We'll have to phone the lab to get the results when the system comes up at ten o'clock." This disconnect between what the physician knows is possible versus what is available at the hospital is putting tremendous pressure on CIOs. And the answers given by CIOs about why this or that can't be done ring hollow. The disconnect creates an even bigger problem for hospital CEOs, planners, and marketers who are trying to build provider networks to maintain volumes. Increasingly they're forced to make promises about ensuring compatibility between computer systems at the hospital and elsewhere that their CIO simply can't deliver in the short term.

Hospitals today must do more with fewer resources if they are to survive. They realize they must increase their investments in computer technology to streamline operations. The stakes are very high. There is little room for error. Management's credibility is on the line in terms of meeting the expectations of patients, their families, their caregivers, and those who pay the bill. It's no wonder health care managers are so concerned with making the right moves when it comes to CIOs and the technology they plan to implement.

The CIO's role is somewhat analogous to the role of the general contractor in the building industry, where the architect (CEO) provides the plans (vision) and the general contractor (CIO) finds the subcontractors (software vendors) to build the building to the customer's (end user's) satisfaction. However, given what's been happening to the health care industry, CIOs who were formerly building pre-fab houses for individual families (information systems for hospitals) have suddenly been thrust into the role of building commercial shopping centers for a multiplicity of uses and customers. The scale of projects is significantly larger, the customers' needs are more diverse, the building codes are more stringent, and the tools and materials and subcontractors are all different.

To be fair, CIOs of large academic medical centers have been building "malls" for years. The problem they now face is to take aging properties and redo them to meet the needs of an upscale clientele with greater expectations about ease of use and service level and to make the change without interrupting service. Some CIOs are up to the task, many are not. This partially explains why many large health care organizations have gone outside the industry to recruit their CIOs. They want someone with a track record of building mega-malls. Each approach has its risks: The CIO with a hospital background may not be up to the task in terms of scale and skill at leading the deployment of new tools and technologies, but the nonhealth care CIO may not be able to cope with the complexity of users' requirements. Neither can survive without unswerving support and sponsorship from the board and CEO.

Although clarity of vision, unswerving sponsorship, and an expert understanding of information technology are necessary components for success, these alone will not meet people's needs. It's the *implementation* of the vision that counts. When it comes to describing the use of technology, *Webster's* the-saurus makes an important contribution. It defines *installation* as *initiation* and *implementation* as *fulfillment.* It is very important to think of technology deployment as a means of fulfilling the needs of the user community. In this era of do more with less, users are redefining their work processes to eliminate waste and increase the focus on outcomes. This process re-design, or reengineering effort, is reaching every area of the health care enterprise. It influences the plan of care by reducing resource consumption and length of stay. It increases patient access and satisfaction and improves clerical productivity and cashflow. Technology must be there to help enable these changes in work process.

It is the health care organization's ability to marry process improvement with technology in a mutually beneficial way that will spell the difference between surviving and thriving. Every health care organization has the same tools available, if not similar resources. Researchers have demonstrated that when organizations fall short in their deployment of technology, it is not usually due to bad planning but rather to poor *execution* of the plan—again, the notion of implementation as fulfillment.

To execute well requires a level of discipline and a structured approach that is missing in many of today's information systems departments. The reliance on vendor-developed software packages in recent years has resulted in atrophy in the ability to design systems. Data processing professionals in health care have become modifiers and maintainers of others' software. They've strayed from their original roles as business analysts and systems designers, and they've become focused on the more nitty-gritty aspects of technical support. Just as it's possible for a radiologist to focus more on the latest image-enhancing technology than on patient needs, so, too, have many information technology professionals become engaged in debating the best database products rather than in finding solutions to users' needs. Meanwhile, Rome is burning.

Fortunately for all concerned, effective implementation of information systems is neither an art form, nor magic, nor even luck. Nor is any invention required in order to be successful. However, it does require a lot of hard work and discipline. It requires power sharing between users and the information systems department so users determine how the systems will function, whereas the information systems department provides a stable, secure platform. The specific choices of computer technology should be transparent to the user, just as the image-compression algorithm of an MRI system is transparent to the patient. This is why information systems departments will require significant increases in capital and operating budgets. They will have to rapidly upgrade the underlying technology infrastructure so they can meet new sets of users needs as required. This technology infrastructure consists of people as well as things. People must have the skills necessary to deal with all the new things that are available and help translate them into solutions for users.

An implementation project has a beginning and an end and must be well managed. A successfully executed project garners executive sponsorship, creates realistic expectations, ensures that appropriate resources are devoted to the project, effectively deals with midstream changes, and provides feedback. No magic. It does, however, require experience. Never use an inexperienced project manager to manage a critical implementation—unless, of course, you want it to take longer than planned, go overbudget, fall short of meeting users needs, or worse yet, crash on takeoff. If you currently have no one with the appropriate level of experience on your staff, hire someone from outside. Hire someone who's done it before and can work well with users. Hire him or her immediately and pay a premium if necessary. This person will provide the leverage for the entire team's success.

By now you should have developed a mental checklist of critical success factors for deploying technology to meet the needs of an integrated health care delivery system. The list should include the following

- Has an information systems plan been developed?

- Does senior management understand and support it?

- Does it support the organization's business strategy?

- Is it realistic? Has it been objectively critiqued?

- Is the chief information officer capable of implementing it?

- Do information systems personnel have the proper skills?

- Do users understand their roles and responsibilities?

- Is there a structured, disciplined approach to implementation?

- Are resources committed and are expectations realistic?

- Is everything about it hospital or acute-care focused?

- Does it take advantage of industry standards?

- Are the expected benefits quantified?

- Are experienced project managers available and committed?

- Is there a way to get timely feedback about progress?

- Is there room for flexibility and changes to the plan?

If you are able to answer yes to all but one of these questions, you have an excellent chance of thriving in the future. If you answer no to more than one of these questions, you have some homework to do. It is hoped this book will provide the reference material you need to deal with this very complex and critical subject.

Index